T0226531

Technology to Assess Sleep

Editor

THOMAS PENZEL

SLEEP MEDICINE CLINICS

www.sleep.theclinics.com

Consulting Editor
TEOFILO LEE-CHIONG Jr

December 2016 • Volume 11 • Number 4

ELSEVIER

1600 John F. Kennedy Boulevard • Suite 1800 • Philadelphia, Pennsylvania, 19103-2899

http://www.theclinics.com

SLEEP MEDICINE CLINICS Volume 11, Number 4
December 2016, ISSN 1556-407X, ISBN-13: 978-0-323-47751-2

Editor: Katie Pfaff
Developmental Editor: Donald Mumford

Sleep Medicine Clinics (ISSN 1556-407X) is published quarterly by Elsevier Inc., 360 Park Avenue South, New York, NY 10010-1710. Months of issue are March, June, September and December. Business and Editorial Offices: 1600 John F. Kennedy Blvd., Ste. 1800, Philadelphia, PA 19103-2899. Customer Service Office: 3251 Riverport Lane, Maryland Heights, MO 63043. Periodicals postage paid at New York, NY and additional mailing offices. Subscription prices are $195.00 per year (US individuals), $100.00 (US students), $458.00 (US institutions), $235.00 (Canadian and international individuals), $135.00 (Canadian and international students), $519.00 (Canadian institutions) and $509.00 (International institutions). Foreign air speed delivery is included in all *Clinics* subscription prices. All prices are subject to change without notice. **POSTMASTER:** Send change of address to *Sleep Medicine Clinics*, Elsevier Health Sciences Division, Subscription Customer Service, 3251 Riverport Lane, Maryland Heights, MO 63043. Customer Service: **Tel: 1-800-654-2452 (U.S. and Canada); 314-447-8871 (outside U.S. and Canada). Fax: 314-447-8029. E-mail: journalscustomerservice-usa@elsevier.com (for print support); journalsonlinesupport-usa@elsevier.com (for online support).**

Reprints. For copies of 100 or more of articles in this publication, please contact the Commercial Reprints Department, Elsevier Inc., 360 Park Avenue South, New York, NY 10010-1710. Tel.: 212-633-3874; Fax: 212-633-3820; E-mail: reprints@elsevier.com.

Sleep Medicine Clinics is covered in *MEDLINE/PubMed (Index Medicus)*.

SLEEP MEDICINE CLINICS

THE CLINICS ARE AVAILABLE ONLINE!
Access your subscription at:
www.theclinics.com

PROGRAM OBJECTIVE

The goal of *Sleep Clinics of North America* is to keep practicing physicians up to date with current clinical practice by providing timely articles reviewing the state of the art in patient care.

TARGET AUDIENCE

All practicing physicians and other healthcare professionals.

LEARNING OBJECTIVES

Upon completion of this activity, participants will be able to:
1. Review emerging technology to assess sleep, such as high-resolution accelerometers and sleep apps.
2. Discuss methods of monitoring sleep-disordered breathing, sleep disturbances with chronic pain, and leg movement activity.
3. Recognize developments in behavioral sleep interventions in pediatrics.

ACCREDITATION

The Elsevier Office of Continuing Medical Education (EOCME) is accredited by the Accreditation Council for Continuing Medical Education (ACCME) to provide continuing medical education for physicians.

The EOCME designates this enduring material for a maximum of 15 *AMA PRA Category 1 Credit*(s)™. Physicians should claim only the credit commensurate with the extent of their participation in the activity.

All other health care professionals requesting continuing education credit for this enduring material will be issued a certificate of participation.

DISCLOSURE OF CONFLICTS OF INTEREST

The EOCME assesses conflict of interest with its instructors, faculty, planners, and other individuals who are in a position to control the content of CME activities. All relevant conflicts of interest that are identified are thoroughly vetted by EOCME for fair balance, scientific objectivity, and patient care recommendations. EOCME is committed to providing its learners with CME activities that promote improvements or quality in healthcare and not a specific proprietary business or a commercial interest.

The planning committee, staff, authors and editors listed below have identified no financial relationships or relationships to products or devices they or their spouse/life partner have with commercial interest related to the content of this CME activity:

Wibke Bartels, MD; Dana Buck, MD; Omar Burschtin, MD; Patjanaporn Chalacheva, PhD; Martin D. Cheatle, PhD; Lara Dhingra, PhD; Raffaele Ferri, MD; Ingo Fietze, MD, PhD; Simmie Foster, MD, PhD; Stephany Fulda, PhD; Martin Glos, MSc; Chantelle N. Hart, PhD; Nicola L. Hawley, PhD; Max Hirshkowitz, PhD; William C. Jangro, DO; Jan W. Kantelhardt, PhD; Michael C.K. Khoo, PhD; Matthew Lesneski, MD; Katie Pfaff; Aaron Pinkett, BS; David Qu, MD; Erin Scheckenbach; Megan Suermann; Rajakumar Venkatesan; Johan Verbraecken, MD, PhD; Jing Wang, MD; Rena R. Wing, PhD; Melanie Zinkhan, PhD.

The planning committee, staff, authors and editors listed below have identified financial relationships or relationships to products or devices they or their spouse/life partner have with commercial interest related to the content of this CME activity:

Erna Sif Arnardottir, PhD is on the speakers' bureau for Weinmann, and is a consultant/advisor for Nox Medical.

Karl Doghramji, MD has stock ownership in Merck & Co., Inc., and is a consultant for Merck & Co., Inc.; Inspire; Jazz Pharmaceuticals; XenoPort, Inc.; Teva Pharmaceutical Industries Ltd; Pfizer Inc; and Pernix Therapeutics.

Thorarinn Gislason, PhD, MD has stock ownership in, and receives lecture fees from, Nox Medical.

Teofilo Lee-Chiong Jr, MD is a consultant/advisor for Elsevier and CareCore International, has stock ownership in and an employment affiliation with Elsevier, and receives royalties/patents from Lippincott; Oxford University Press; CreateSpace; and Wiley.

Thomas Penzel, PhD has research support from Koninklijke Philips N.V.; ResMed; Itamar Medical Ltd; Cidelec; Nomics s.a.; and Weinmann Geräte für Medizin GmbH + Co. KG.

UNAPPROVED/OFF-LABEL USE DISCLOSURE

The EOCME requires CME faculty to disclose to the participants:
1. When products or procedures being discussed are off-label, unlabelled, experimental, and/or investigational (not US Food and Drug Administration [FDA] approved); and
2. Any limitations on the information presented, such as data that are preliminary or that represent ongoing research, interim analyses, and/or unsupported opinions. Faculty may discuss information about pharmaceutical agents that is outside of FDA-approved labelling. This information is intended solely for CME and is not intended to promote off-label use of these medications. If you have any questions, contact the medical affairs department of the manufacturer for the most recent prescribing information.

TO ENROLL

To enroll in the Sleep Medicines Clinic Continuing Medical Education program, call customer service at 1-800-654-2452 or sign up online at http://www.theclinics.com/home/cme. The CME program is available to subscribers for an additional annual fee of USD $140.

METHOD OF PARTICIPATION

In order to claim credit, participants must complete the following:

1. Complete enrolment as indicated above.
2. Read the activity.
3. Complete the CME Test and Evaluation. Participants must achieve a score of 70% on the test. All CME Tests and Evaluations must be completed online.

CME INQUIRIES/SPECIAL NEEDS

For all CME inquiries or special needs, please contact elsevierCME@elsevier.com.

Contributors

CONSULTING EDITOR

TEOFILO LEE-CHIONG Jr, MD
Professor of Medicine, National Jewish Health;
Professor of Medicine, School of Medicine,
University of Colorado Denver, Denver,
Colorado; Chief Medical Liaison, Philips
Respironics, Pennsylvania

EDITOR

THOMAS PENZEL, PhD
Scientific Director of Sleep Center,
Interdisciplinary Center of Sleep Medicine,
Department of Cardiology, Charité
Universitätsmedizin Berlin, Berlin, Germany;
Senior Researcher, International Clinical
Research Center, St. Anne's University
Hospital Brno, Brno, Czech Republic

AUTHORS

ERNA SIF ARNARDOTTIR, PhD
Director of Sleep Measurements,
Department of Respiratory Medicine and
Sleep, Landspitali – The National University
Hospital of Iceland; Postdoctoral Researcher,
Faculty of Medicine, University of Iceland,
Reykjavik, Iceland

WIBKE BARTELS, MD
Interdisciplinary Center of Sleep Medicine,
Department of Cardiology, Charité
Universitätsmedizin Berlin, Berlin, Germany

DANA BUCK, MD
Interdisciplinary Center of Sleep Medicine,
Department of Cardiology; Department of
Oto-Rhino-Laryngology, Charité
Universitätsmedizin Berlin, Berlin, Germany

OMAR BURSCHTIN, MD
Division of Pulmonary, Critical Care and
Sleep Medicine, Associate Professor,
Mount Sinai School of Medicine, New York,
New York

PATJANAPORN CHALACHEVA, PhD
Research Associate, Biomedical Engineering
Department, University of Southern California,
Los Angeles, California

MARTIN D. CHEATLE, PhD
Center for Studies of Addiction, Perelman
School of Medicine, University of
Pennsylvania, Philadelphia, Pennsylvania;
Reading Health System, West Reading,
Pennsylvania

LARA DHINGRA, PhD
MJHS Institute for Innovation in Palliative Care,
New York, New York

KARL DOGHRAMJI, MD
Professor of Psychiatry, Neurology, and
Medicine; Program Director, Fellowship in
Sleep Medicine, Department of Psychiatry and
Human Behavior; Medical Director, Jefferson
Sleep Disorders Center, Sidney Kimmel
Medical College, Thomas Jefferson University,
Philadelphia, Pennsylvania

RAFFAELE FERRI, MD
Department of Neurology I.C., Senior Staff
Specialist; Head, Sleep Research Centre, Oasi
Institute for Research on Mental Retardation
and Brain Aging (IRCCS), Troina, Italy

INGO FIETZE, MD, PhD
Interdisciplinary Center of Sleep Medicine,
Department of Cardiology, Charité
Universitätsmedizin Berlin, Berlin, Germany

SIMMIE FOSTER, MD, PhD
Kirby Center for Neurobiology, Boston,
Massachusetts

STEPHANY FULDA, PhD
Neurocenter of Southern Switzerland, Sleep
and Epilepsy Center, Civic Hospital (EOC) of
Lugano, Lugano, Switzerland

THORARINN GISLASON, PhD, MD
Chief, Department of Respiratory Medicine and
Sleep, Landspitali – The National University
Hospital of Iceland; Professor, Faculty of
Medicine, University of Iceland, Reykjavik,
Iceland

MARTIN GLOS, MSc
Interdisciplinary Center of Sleep Medicine,
Department of Cardiology, Charité
Universitätsmedizin Berlin, Berlin, Germany

CHANTELLE N. HART, PhD
Associate Professor, Department of Social and
Behavioral Sciences, Center for Obesity
Research and Education, College of Public
Health, Temple University, Philadelphia,
Pennsylvania

NICOLA L. HAWLEY, PhD
Assistant Professor, Department of Chronic
Disease Epidemiology, Yale School of Public
Health, New Haven, Connecticut

MAX HIRSHKOWITZ, PhD
Consulting Professor, Division of Public Mental
Health and Population Sciences, School of
Medicine, Stanford University, Palo Alto,
California; Full Professor (Emeritus),
Department of Medicine, Baylor College of
Medicine, Houston, Texas

WILLIAM C. JANGRO, DO
Assistant Professor of Psychiatry; Associate
Director, Adult Residency Training Program,
Department of Psychiatry and Human
Behavior, Sidney Kimmel Medical College,
Thomas Jefferson University, Philadelphia,
Pennsylvania

JAN W. KANTELHARDT, PhD
Institute of Physics, Faculty of Natural
Sciences II, Martin-Luther-University Halle-
Wittenberg, Halle; Cardiovascular Physics,
Department of Physics, Humboldt-University
of Berlin, Berlin, Germany

MICHAEL C.K. KHOO, PhD
Professor of Biomedical Engineering and
Pediatrics, Biomedical Engineering
Department, University of Southern California,
Los Angeles, California

MATTHEW LESNESKI, MD
RA Pain Services, Mount Laurel, New Jersey

THOMAS PENZEL, PhD
Scientific Director of Sleep Center,
Interdisciplinary Center of Sleep Medicine,
Department of Cardiology, Charité
Universitätsmedizin Berlin, Berlin, Germany;
Senior Researcher, International Clinical
Research Center, St. Anne's University
Hospital Brno, Brno, Czech Republic

AARON PINKETT, BS
Center for Studies of Addiction, Perelman
School of Medicine, University of
Pennsylvania, Philadelphia, Pennsylvania

DAVID QU, MD
Highpoint Pain and Rehabilitation Physicians
P.C., Chalfont, Pennsylvania

JOHAN VERBRAECKEN, MD, PhD
Department of Pulmonary Medicine,
Multidisciplinary Sleep Disorders Centre,
Antwerp University Hospital, University of
Antwerp, Edegem, Antwerp, Belgium

JING WANG, MD
Division of Pulmonary, Critical Care, and Sleep
Medicine, Sleep Medicine Fellow, NYU School
of Medicine, New York, New York

RENA R. WING, PhD
Professor, Department of Psychiatry and
Human Behavior, Weight Control and Diabetes
Research Center, The Miriam Hospital, Alpert
Medical School of Brown University,
Providence, Rhode Island

MELANIE ZINKHAN, PhD
Institute of Medical Epidemiology,
Biostatistics and Informatics,
Faculty of Medicine, Martin-Luther-University
Halle-Wittenberg, Halle,
Germany

Contents

Polysomnography provided a means to objectively study sleep. Initial challenges were technical; the next challenge was overcoming communication difficulties and lack of standardization. The new specialty, sleep medicine, created a huge demand for laboratory polysomnography. By the early 2000s, home sleep testing and treatment devices made inroads into clinical sleep practice. The economic consequence was shrinking demand for clinical laboratory polysomnography. Therefore, polysomnography must now find new directions, approaches, and purpose. Engineering challenges remain, and the "new" polysomnography needs to revisit some of the original questions about sleep, including what constitutes optimal sleep quantity, timing, and quality.

Currently, 2 sets of similar rules for recording and scoring leg movement (LM) exist, including periodic LM during sleep (PLMS) and periodic LM during wakefulness. The former were published in 2006 by a task force of the International Restless Legs Syndrome Study Group, and the second in 2007 by the American Academy of Sleep Medicine. This article reviews the basic recording methods, scoring rules, and computer-based programs for PLMS. Less frequent LM activities, such as alternating leg muscle activation, hypnagogic foot tremor, high-frequency LMs, and excessive fragmentary myoclonus are briefly described.

Traditional techniques to assess respiratory disturbances during sleep allow the accurate diagnosis of moderate and severe cases of obstructive sleep apnea but have serious limitations in mild obstructive sleep apnea and cases with signs of obstructive breathing during sleep without apneas and hypopneas. This article describes advantages and limitations of available techniques to measure obstructive breathing during sleep by measuring flow limitation, respiratory effort, and snoring. Standardization of these techniques is crucial for moving the field further and understanding the pathophysiologic role of obstructive breathing itself, and not solely focusing on the associated outcomes of arousals and oxygen desaturations.

Model-Derived Markers of Autonomic Cardiovascular Dysfunction in Sleep-Disordered Breathing   489

Michael C.K. Khoo and Patjanaporn Chalacheva

Evidence indicates that sleep-disordered breathing leads to elevated sympathetic tone and impaired vagal activity, promoting hypertension and cardiometabolic disease. Low-cost but accurate monitoring of autonomic function is useful for the aggressive management of sleep apnea. This article reviews the development and application of multivariate dynamic biophysical models that enable the causal dependencies among respiration, blood pressure, heart rate variability, and peripheral vascular resistance to be quantified. The markers derived from these models can be used in conjunction with heart rate variability to increase the sensitivity with which abnormalities in autonomic cardiovascular control are detected in subjects with sleep-disordered breathing.

Special Articles

Adverse Effects of Psychotropic Medications on Sleep   503

Karl Doghramji and William C. Jangro

Psychotropic medications such as antidepressants, antipsychotics, stimulants, and benzodiazepines are widely prescribed. Most of these medications are thought to exert their effects through modulation of various monoamines as well as interactions with receptors such as histamine and muscarinic cholinergic receptors. Through these interactions, psychotropics can also have a significant impact on sleep physiology, resulting in both beneficial and adverse effects on sleep.

Development of a Behavioral Sleep Intervention as a Novel Approach for Pediatric Obesity in School-aged Children   515

Chantelle N. Hart, Nicola L. Hawley, and Rena R. Wing

Despite being the focus of widespread public health efforts, childhood obesity remains an epidemic worldwide. Given the now well-documented consequences of obesity for childhood health and psychosocial functioning, as well as associated morbidity in adulthood, identifying novel, modifiable behaviors that can be targeted to improve weight control is imperative. Enhancing children's sleep may show promise in assisting with weight regulation. The present paper describes the development of a brief behavioral sleep intervention for school-aged children, including preliminary findings of this work as well as areas for future study.

Testosterone Deficiency and Sleep Apnea   525

Omar Burschtin and Jing Wang

Obstructive sleep apnea (OSA) is a common condition among middle-aged men and is often associated with reduced testosterone (T) levels. OSA can contribute to fatigue and sexual dysfunction in men. There is suggestion that T supplementation alters ventilatory responses, possibly through effects on central chemoreceptors. Traditionally, it has been recommended that T replacement therapy (TRT) be avoided in the presence of untreated severe sleep apnea. With OSA treatment, however, TRT may not only improve hypogonadism, but may also alleviate erectile/sexual dysfunction.

Assessing and Managing Sleep Disturbance in Patients with Chronic Pain   531

Martin D. Cheatle, Simmie Foster, Aaron Pinkett, Matthew Lesneski, David Qu, and Lara Dhingra

Chronic pain is associated with symptoms that may impair a patient's quality of life, including emotional distress, fatigue, and sleep disturbance. There is a high prevalence of concomitant pain and sleep disturbance. Studies support the hypothesis that sleep and pain have a bidirectional and reciprocal relationship. Clinicians who manage patients with chronic pain often focus on interventions that relieve pain, and assessing and treating sleep disturbance are secondary or not addressed. This article reviews the literature on pain and co-occurring sleep disturbance, describes the assessment of sleep disturbance, and outlines nonpharmacologic and pharmacologic treatment strategies to improve sleep in patients with chronic pain.

Preface
Current State and Future Perspectives for the Assessment of Sleep Using Modern Technology

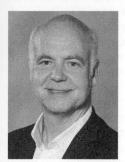

Thomas Penzel, PhD

Editor

Sleep medicine and sleep research are medical fields with much modern technology involved. The development of sleep medicine and sleep research is closely linked to the development of the investigational tool, polysomnography, as outlined in much more detail by Dr Hirshkowitz (see article, "Polysomnography Challenges"). However, becoming more clinical, the field of sleep medicine went far beyond quantitative sleep investigations in a protected and supervised room. Much of sleep medicine today is performed by careful interviews and clinical investigations. Sleep medicine no longer means investigations during sleep alone; it includes investigations during the daytime in order to check for the results of restorative sleep. With the increasing number of sleep and wakefulness complaints, the number of patients suffering is increasing dramatically. Our knowledge about sleep disorders helped to identify how far some disorders can be diagnosed at home using out-of-center technology. As a young, emerging, and interdisciplinary field of modern medicine, this arena is particularly open to new technologies. Sleep medicine today makes use of advanced computer programs in the diagnosis of sleep disorders, in applying telemedicine communication technologies, and in reaching out to smartphone-based applications (apps) for the diagnosis or diagnostic support of assessing sleep disorders. Dr Ferri uses modern

signal processing technologies to support computer-based analysis of movement disorders during sleep (see article, "Quantifying Leg Movement Activity During Sleep"). The article shows very well that computer-based analysis has limited applicability when definitions are fuzzy or contradictive. A similar problem occurs in the quantification of airflow limitation and snoring for sleep-related breathing disorders (see article, "Quantifying Airflow Limitation and Snoring During Sleep," by Dr Arnardottir). Finally, most sleep disorders show, as a common mechanism, central nervous arousal, which disturbs sleep. The big question for pathophysiology to clarify is, how far does arousal cause cardiovascular consequences? There a quantitative assessment of cortical, and subcortical, or heart rate and blood pressure–mediated arousal is needed (see article, "Definition and Importance of Autonomic Arousal in Patients with Sleep Disordered Breathing," by Dr Bartels). Computer-based methods may help to assess autonomic arousal quantitatively and reliable in the future. Many sleep disorders are chronic disorders. Sleep apnea as one important problem with a high prevalence not only needs an initial diagnosis but also follow-up studies, which cannot be performed by in-lab studies due to quantity. Here, telemedicine apps offer options for the long-term follow-up of our patients (see article, "Telemedicine Applications in Sleep

Sleep Med Clin 11 (2016) xv–xvi
http://dx.doi.org/10.1016/j.jsmc.2016.09.001
1556-407X/16/© 2016 Published by Elsevier Inc.

Disordered Breathing Thinking Out of the Box," by Dr Verbraecken). Because sleep complaints are gaining more public awareness, smartphone apps, which support the "quantify yourself" movement, added sleep as a popular and economically important field. Here, the borders between medical diagnosis and assessing well-being (who bears the costs?) are still undefined. This emerging field is reviewed by Dr Fietze (see article, "Sleep Applications to Assess Sleep Quality"). With the limited clinical sleep centers in place and the increasing number of sleep apps, the uncertainty, of how prevalent sleep disorders are, increases. And in how far sleep disorders are linked to morbidity and mortality. For some disorders, like obstructive sleep apnea, such studies are available; for most studies, this is not the case. And therefore, we need good and carefully planned epidemiologic studies that assess sleep with adequate and low-cost tools (see article, "Sleep Assessment in Large Cohort Studies with High-Resolution Accelerometers," by Dr Zinkhan). Epidemiology is one end of research where technology can help. Physiology and pathophysiologic mechanisms are the other end of the research strip. Therefore, this issue is

concluded with a research article that explains how technical developments are used to model disorder mechanisms and thereby allow a better understanding and potentially a better treatment (see article, "Model-Derived Markers of Autonomic Cardiovascular Dysfunction in Sleep-Disordered Breathing," by Dr Khoo). For this approach, new markers of autonomic cardiovascular dysfunction in sleep apnea are derived and presented by Dr Khoo. Altogether, new technical developments advance the field of sleep research and sleep medicine in many diverse aspects. Imaging, genetics, biomarkers, and pharmaceutical and therapeutic methods were not even touched in this issue and should be covered in future.

Thomas Penzel, PhD
Scientific Director of Sleep Center
Interdisciplinary Center of Sleep Medicine
Department of Cardiology
Charité Universitätsmedizin Berlin
Charitéplatz 1
10117 Berlin, Germany

E-mail address:
Thomas.penzel@charite.de

Polysomnography Challenges

Max Hirshkowitz, PhD[a,b,*]

KEYWORDS

- Polysomnography • Sleep studies • Sleep evaluation • Sleep medicine • Home sleep testing

KEY POINTS

- Polysomnography began as a tool of discovery, but its primary use quickly evolved into a clinical procedure for diagnosing sleep disorders.
- Diagnosis and treatment of sleep disorders created a huge demand for clinical polysomnographic services. However, by the early 2000s, outpatient testing and treatment reduced this demand for clinical laboratory polysomnography in favor of other methods.
- Current engineering challenges include using wireless technology, less intrusive measures, new biomedical sensors, and a "big data" analytical approach to reinvent polysomnography. This new polysomnography may tell us what constitutes optimal sleep quantity, timing, and quality.

THE CHALLENGES: OVERVIEW

To study sleep objectively, polysomnography provided a means. It was a tool of discovery born into the golden age of physiology. Once under way, there were technical challenges to overcome related to recording, data reduction, and information processing. Notions about where discovery's fertile ground might be located guided recording channel selection. Psychophysiologists, who are notorious tool makers, in concert with bioengineers, seized the opportunity, improved on, and applied many new techniques. Indeed, the original sleep research society was called The Association for the Psychophysiological Study of Sleep. As often happens when a field expands rapidly, data were (1) collected using different procedures, (2) described using idiosyncratic terminology, and (3) summarized in different ways. Difficulty comparing results from different laboratories presented another challenge. The solution was standardization; however, standardization can be a double-edged sword inasmuch as it can both facilitate progress and stifle creative advance.

Clinical researchers quickly realized polysomnography's potential in biomedical applications. This helped create a new medical specialty: sleep medicine. The discovery that sleep-related breathing disorders are both common and medically serious contributed largely to polysomnography's primary application becoming sleep apnea diagnosis. Furthermore, an effective noninvasive treatment was found that could be titrated during concurrent polysomnographic (ie, positive airway pressure therapy). Coupled together, these 2 discoveries fueled sleep medicine's rapid growth. As a result, the challenge became one of meeting demand for diagnostic and treatment services.

Polysomnography, however, being born in the research laboratory as a tool for discovery, is not necessarily the most efficient tool for diagnostic verification. Miniaturization, new biomedical sensor technology, digital amplifier advances, and more sophisticated computer applications marched forward. Home sleep-testing devices and self-titrating positive airway pressure devices steadily improved. As medical practice began to

Disclosure Statement: The author has nothing to disclose.
[a] Division of Public Mental Health and Population Sciences, School of Medicine, Stanford University, 3430 Bayshore Road, Palo Alto, CA 94303, USA; [b] Department of Medicine, Baylor College of Medicine, 1 Baylor Plaza, Houston, TX 77030, USA
* Corresponding author. 4380 Vine Hill Road, Sebastopol, CA 95472.
E-mail address: max.hirshkowitz@gmail.com

Sleep Med Clin 11 (2016) 403–411
http://dx.doi.org/10.1016/j.jsmc.2016.07.002
1556-407X/16/© 2016 Elsevier Inc. All rights reserved.

apply these advanced technologies, the demand for diagnostic polysomnographic services slowed and began to decline. This winnowing continues to generate a retooling challenge as sleep medicine (and polysomnography) must change with the times, least it perish.

The challenge now facing polysomnography involves the search for new directions. Polysomnography began in the analog age and transitioned by having digital technology simulate earlier analog equipment. Some of the current engineering challenges involve incorporating wireless technology, integrating newer biomedical sensors, coordinating data gathered from multiple sources, developing less intrusive measurement devices, and coordinating large data arrays for tracking data over extended time periods. From a scientific perspective, revisiting the original questions about sleep's nature and function remains the ultimate challenge. An updated and modernized version of polysomnography may provide answers to our questions concerning optimal sleep quantity, timing, and quality.

OBJECTIVELY STUDYING SLEEP

The term polysomnography identifies a method developed to physiologically describe human sleep. It was used to provide scientific information beyond what Kleitman[1] had designated the "basic rest activity cycle." Polysomnography began as an application of electrophysiological technology. The initial electrophysiological description of sleep came from Hans Berger,[2] the father of electroencephalography (EEG). Almost 90 years ago, Berger[2] recorded a single EEG channel and found alpha activity disappearance correlated with self-reported perception of being asleep. However, the Loomis research group,[3] conducting research at the Tuxedo Park Laboratories in the late 1930s, published the first account of continuous, all-night, multiple-channel, sleep recordings. These recordings arguably represent the initial primordial version of the procedure that ultimately became polysomnography.

The Tuxedo Park recordings consisted of simultaneous ink-on-paper tracings of activity from 3 derivations, selectable between midline vertex, midline occiput, behind left and right ears, and just above and to the left of the left eye. A fourth channel could be used for recording either signal markers, heartbeats, or respiration. The investigators noted general activity pattern clusters that changed suddenly. From this observation, they described specific *states of sleep and wakefulness*, labeling them stage A, B, C, D, and E. Interestingly, although an electrode was positioned such that it could record eye movement, no mention of rapid eye movement during "activated" or "light" sleep was made even though dreaming reportedly occurred during a type of sleep designated as stage B. Nonetheless, the Tuxedo Group clearly identified multiple processes ongoing during sleep that recurred in an orderly, regular sequence. Furthermore, brain activity was clearly the group's focus.

The electrophysiological description of sleep advanced about a decade and a half later when Eugene Aserisky and his mentor Nathanial Kleitman[4] correlated EEG activity accompanied by jerky eye movements with dreaming. Kleitman had already previously regrouped sleep into stages 1, 2, 3, and 4 based on brainwave patterns. The sleep stage containing this additional feature (rapid eye movements) ultimately became known as rapid eye movement (REM) sleep (although other names were initially used). This discovery captured the imagination of many psychiatrically minded researchers for, as Kleitman[1] put it in his book *Sleep and Wakefulness*, "...we literally stumbled on an objective method of studying dreaming...."

STANDARDIZATION

Within another decade and a half, an ad hoc committee met and eventually agreed to standardize recording techniques, methods, and nomenclature to aid scientific communication and facilitate sleep research.[5] Several sleep scoring systems had evolved and each used different time domains, criteria, and summarization rules. Furthermore, an assortment of terms for essentially the same phenomena were in use. For example, REM sleep was also called paradoxic sleep, desynchronized sleep, active sleep, D sleep, and even unorthodox sleep, depending on where the research was conducted. The resultant standardization defined polysomnography for research applications. Recommended recordings included an EEG recorded from a central derivation, electrooculograms (EOG) from the right and left eye, and a surface electrode electromyogram recorded near the chin (EMG submentalis). The EMG submentalis was included because Jouvet and Michel[6] had found loss of muscle tone during REM sleep in cats and this phenomenon also occurred in humans. The published description of this standard technique is often called *The R&K Manual* (referring to the committee chairmen Allan Rechtschaffen and Anthony Kales). The standardization effort succeeded largely because consensus was reached. Researchers went back to their laboratories and began using the standardized system. Many quickly began comparing biological and mental phenomena during REM sleep with other sleep stages. Others examined age and sex differences. Finally, sleep was poked and prodded by deprivation, drugs, and environmental/behavioral manipulations to see how it responded. Standardization certainly facilitated communication.

Although not part of the standard, the workhorse apparatus in many laboratories became the Grass model 78 EEG machine adapted for polysomnography (**Figs. 1** and **2**). Additionally, advances in quantitative methods, analytical techniques, and sensor technology, spurred on sleep research. Ultimately, analog amplifiers gave way to digital recording technology. The era of ink-stained laboratory coats and fan-fold paper stacked against walls and in storage rooms slowly disappeared. The newer digital technology allowed users to change time constants, temporal resolution, bandpass filtering, amplitude gain, and recording channel arrays after the fact. Polysomnographers are not nostalgic about pen blocking, ink spattering, paper cuts, and piles of paper adorning their offices and laboratories (**Figs. 3** and **4**).

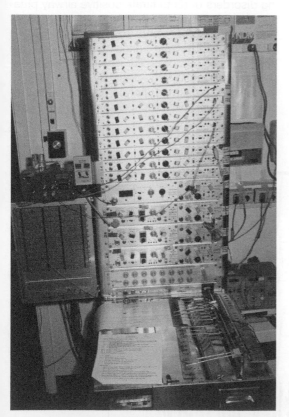

Fig. 1. Grass model 78 EEG machine adapted for polysomnographic recording.

Early attempts at computerizing polysomnography focused on sleep stage and polysomnographic event scoring. To anyone involved in the summary of all-night continuous sleep studies, the time intensiveness required for scoring was painfully obvious. Large-scale overhead mass storage devices, suitable computer-processing speeds, and adequate random access memory arrays were not yet available for laboratory computers. Consequently, alternate processing strategies emerged. One approach to solving these problems involved simultaneously recording the entire study on analog tape and playing it back into the computer offline. Tapes could be digitized at high speed or pre-processed with bandpass separations for sleep staging (for example, Jack Smith's Sleep Analyzing Hybrid Computer system). Analog instrument tape recorders, however, were extremely expensive (eg, Ampex FR1300 [Redwood City, CA], Sangamo Sabre II [Springfield, IL], and Hewlett-Packard 7470 recorders [Palo Alto, CA]). Another approach used pre-processing with scoring and compression in real time (eg, Vitalog [Redwood City, CA]). Such systems did not always retain the actual raw data so validation could be difficult (if not impossible). Over time, small computer capabilities caught up to researcher's desires. Ironically, once microcomputer systems became fast enough, equipped with adequate memory, and affordable, they were mainly used to replace paper (and its accompanying costs for purchase, handling, and storage). Well-validated automatic scoring for sleep stages and accompanying events continued unrealized for more than 2 decades and some would argue remains so today. In part, the reason for this stemmed from the polysomnographic applications' global change in direction and purpose.

SLEEP MEDICINE RISING

Perhaps the greatest catalyst propelling the polysomnography juggernaut was the potential for biomedical applications. During the decade following standardization, clinical researchers identified several, rather unique, medical sleep-related pathophysiologies.[7] Recordings of respiration, heart rhythm, and movements during sleep inexorably lead what we now call *clinical polysomnography*. Most notably, breathing and movement disorders associated with sleep. More refined methods developed to identify these disorders and clinical polysomnography began to take shape. The methods described in Christian Guilleminault's[8] *Sleeping and Waking Disorders: Indications and Techniques* essentially became the *defacto standard* for extending polysomnography beyond the *R&K Manual* for

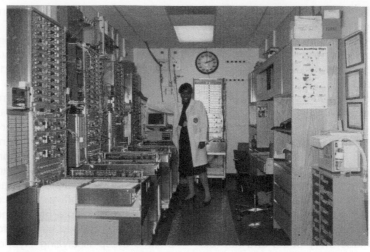

Fig. 2. Sleep laboratory control room, circa 1979.

clinical purposes. It was finally superseded in 2007 when the American Academy of Sleep Medicine (AASM) published its standardized manual for using polysomnography in sleep medicine.[9]

In addition to its use in research applications, polysomnography acquired clinical indications for diagnosing sleep-related breathing disorders, titrating positive airway pressure for treating sleep-related breathing disorders, identifying periodic limb movement disorder, confirming narcolepsy, and differentiating parasomnias from nocturnal seizures.[10] Additional applications included diagnosing insomnia, differentiating psychogenic from organic erectile dysfunction, and

searching for any EEG, electrocardiographic, or physiologic abnormality to help elucidate difficult, puzzling sleep disorder cases.

As a practical matter, however, the *vast* majority of clinical polysomnographic recordings were made to either (1) diagnose sleep-related breathing disorders or (2) to titrate positive airway pressure.[11] Conservatively, more than 80% of all polysomnographic sleep studies performed in the past decade were conducted for one or the other of these purposes. Parasomnias are rare disorders that are mainly diagnosed clinically but sometimes confirmed polysomnographically. In some countries, narcolepsy diagnosis may involve

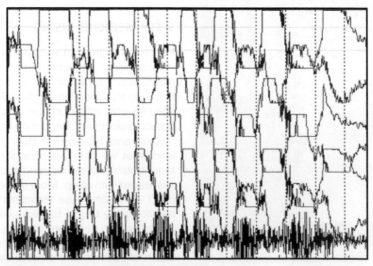

Fig. 3. Pen blocking during polysomnographic recording.

polysomnography conducted for another purpose. Thus, in California Silicon Valley techie jargon, polysomnography has become the "killer app" for diagnosing sleep apnea.

Sleep disorders centers and sleep-disordered breathing diagnostic units sprang up in medical schools, hospitals, and as free-standing laboratories. In the United States, significant infrastructure grew and by 2013 there were 2500 AASM-accredited facilities.[12] No accurate count of nonaccredited sleep disorders units is available; however, it is likely some substantial multiple of the AASM tally. Digital polysomnographic equipment, positive airway pressure machine, and pulse oximeter manufacturing became big businesses. Smaller enterprises producing and distributing electrodes, biosensors, and other ancillary equipment were also lifted on the incoming tide targeting clinical applications. **Fig. 5** illustrates the development and expansion of polysomnographic applications from descriptive research to clinical research and from clinical research to clinical practice. The main challenge during this expansion period was keeping pace with the demand for clinical services. This was especially true for public health care institutions whose available resources were already overburdened.

THE WINNOWING

As health care costs grow, several economic-related challenges arise. First, institutions and

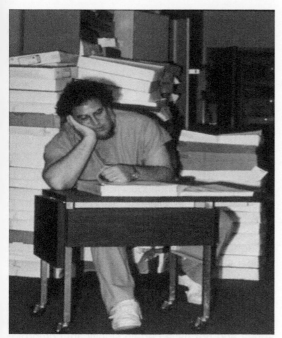

Fig. 4. Author surrounded by a sea of paper polysomnograms.

overnight polysomnography followed the next day by a multiple sleep latency test. However, narcolepsy too is a relatively rare disorder compared with sleep apnea. Periodic limb movement disorder is often clear from the history (especially if the bed partner is available for interview) or is discovered as an incidental finding during

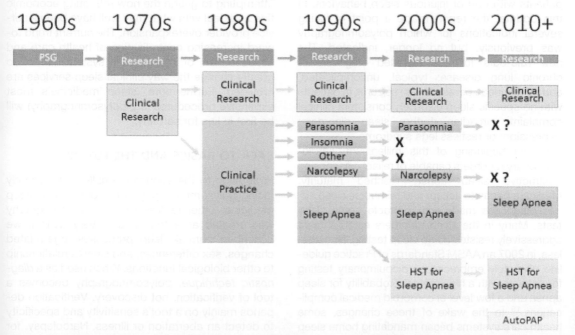

Fig. 5. A timeline of polysomnography expansion and contraction in the past 50+ years. AutoPAP, automatically self-adjusting positive airway pressure device; HST, home sleep testing; PSG, polysomnography.

insurers increase their scrutiny of budgets, especially for high line-item expenditures. To justify (and possibly streamline) medical practice, professional organizations sometimes issue *standards of practice guidelines* using evidence-based medicine to substantiate their recommendations. Additionally, new technologies offering alternative approaches (and invariably promising greater cost-effectiveness), find such conditions an opportunity for growth. All 3 of these factors represent current challenges for clinical polysomnography.

In 1997, the AASM provided practice parameters for clinical polysomnography.[10] The recommended indications for sleep studies were based on peer-reviewed literature evidence and a consensus of a task force convened for that purpose. The AASM Board of Directors then modified and endorsed the guidelines. In 2005, these practice parameters were updated by the AASM Standards of Practice Committee using a modified Sackett (1993)[13] evidence-based medicine approach.[14] Decisions in areas in which there was insufficient available evidence, a RAND appropriateness method was used to reach consensus for clinical recommendations. The indications for polysomnography were trimmed to include diagnosing sleep apnea, periodic limb movement disorder, and narcolepsy. Sleep studies also were recommended for titrating positive airway pressure in patients with sleep apnea and for identifying nocturnal seizure disorders in patients with odd or injurious sleep behaviors. In this update, the report made a point of listing several indications for which polysomnography was previously, but no longer, indicated. The new rule-outs for use included diagnosis of chronic lung disease; typical, uncomplicated, and noninjurious parasomnias; seizures in patients with no specific sleep disorder, consistent clinical complaint; circadian rhythm sleep disorders; depression; or restless legs syndrome.

At the beginning of this millennium, cardiopulmonary recorders capable of reliably diagnosing obstructive sleep apnea reached maturity. Medicare began to accept and reimburse sleep apnea diagnoses made with portable home sleep tests. Many in the sleep disorders establishment aggressively resisted home sleep testing. Nonetheless, in 2007 an AASM Standards of Practice guideline ultimately embraced cardiopulmonary testing for patients with a high pretest probability for sleep apnea and a low level of comorbid medical complications.[15] In the wake of these changes, some health care systems began mandating home sleep testing as a first-line approach for diagnosing sleep-related breathing disorders.

In approximately the same time frame during which home cardiopulmonary recorders were gaining acceptance, automatic self-titrating positive airway pressure machines (APAP) appeared on the market. These devices monitored airflow, pressure, vibration, and/or volume and adjusted positive pressure in an attempt to normalize breathing. In theory, these machines could perform titration. In 2002, based on a thorough clinical literature review, the AASM Standards of Practice Committee concluded "Use of unattended APAP to either initially determine pressures for fixed CPAP [continuous positive airway pressure] or for self-adjusting APAP treatment in CPAP-naïve patients is not currently established."[16] However, within the next 5 years, enough literature accrued to update the AASM clinical guideline to approve using unattended APAP machines as a clinical option to determine positive airway pressure, with certain restrictions.[17] The restrictions were that the patient must have moderate or severe obstructive sleep apnea and not have certain significant comorbidities (central sleep apnea, hypoventilation syndromes, congestive heart failure, of chronic obstructive pulmonary disease).

These 2 technologies (cardiopulmonary recorders and APAP) combined with a winnowing of practice parameters recommending in-laboratory sleep studies, portended slowing growth and eventually a shrinking market for polysomnography (**Fig. 6**). The challenge at this point is attempting to gauge the now retreating economic tide and deal with what may well have been a service provider overexpansion. The current trend toward increasing centralization of health care and consolidation of health care systems will also greatly change the way clinical sleep services are provided. Furthermore, sleep medicine's most expensive procedures (eg, polysomnography) will be first in line for scrutiny.

BACK TO BASICS AND THE FUTURE

In addition to the economic challenges currently facing polysomnography in the practice of sleep medicine, other factors exist. Polysomnography was created as a tool of discovery. With it we described normal sleep processes, age-related changes, sex differences, and sleep's relationship to other biological functions. When used as a *diagnostic technique*, polysomnography becomes a tool of verification, not discovery. Verification depends mainly on a tool's sensitivity and specificity to detect an aberration or illness. Narcolepsy, for example, can now be verified using cerebrospinal fluid. At some point in the future, it is conceivable

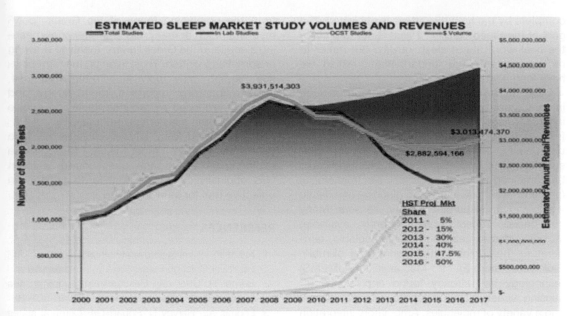

Fig. 6. Changes in the clinical use of polysomnography and predicted trends from T. Crabtree of Health Strategy Partners. (*From* Crabtree T. Sleep 2014 what to expect – how to prepare. Presented at The Business of Sleep October 29 & 30, 2014, Bear Mountain, NY. Health Strategy Partners. Available at: foocus.com/power-point/Sleep-in-2014-and-beyond.pdf. Accessed June 6, 2016; with permission.)

that narcolepsy, and possibly other sleep disorders, will be diagnosed with a blood or DNA test. The trend in medical practice is away from complex, time-consuming tests and toward specimen analysis or image scans.

The current challenge for polysomnography is to innovate, advance, and reposition itself as a relevant method for understanding processes underlying sleep. Is it possible that polysomnography's meteoric rise and early success, stifled innovation? Were our forbearers in sleep research so brilliant that they devised a near perfect system from the very start? Or have we gotten complacent? Indeed, the basic recording approach for sleep studies has changed little in the past 30 years. Reviewing a clinical polysomnogram may have changed platforms (from ink on paper to pixels on a screen) but the content analysis remains quite similar. This is perhaps even more ironic given the enormous computing power built into the machines that we use chiefly as recorder-displayer-summarizers. My colleague, Dr Sassin chuckles when he points out that we can wirelessly deliver heart, respiratory, and oxyhemoglobin signals from earth-orbiting spacecraft but we still attach wires, sit in the adjoining room, and manually score sleep recordings.

To be fair, however, we have been able to extract more information from polysomnographic recordings than in the past. Understanding how brief central nervous system arousals alter sleep's restorative processes provided insight into the sleep process.[18] The attention to and quantification of sleep-related cyclic alternating patterns[19] brought a new appreciation for the need for a dynamic sleep model. Pulse wave analysis and cardiopulmonary coupling exemplify the power of advanced analytical techniques for extracting additional information from recordings. Such advances harken back to the spirit of applied methodology for advancing the field and possibly making discovery.

One longstanding scientific challenge for polysomnography has been to define normal sleep and sleep quality. Good-quality sleep is the foundation for health (along with nutrition and exercise). Overall, *sleep health* includes sleep quantity, sleep quality, sleep timing, satisfaction with sleep, and absence of sleep disorders. Sleep disorders potentially impair any or all of the aforementioned sleep health elements and, as such, dominated polysomnographic applications. We require sleep to perform 3 basic functions: garbage collection (removal of toxins), material resupply (restocking of neurochemicals and other humors), and growth. Nonetheless, defining sleep quality is a daunting task. Quality invariably combines different components in a way that optimizes or improves a material or process's worth. As the current chairman, I urged the National Sleep Foundation to sponsor a renewed attempt to define sleep quality based on polysomnography. This process is currently under way and may be complete by the time this article is published. The goal of the Sleep Quality Project is not to provide the final word about sleep quality, but rather to reopen interest in a fundamental question we have long neglected.

Other challenges for polysomnography include integrating advances in sensor technology, making recordings wireless, and integrating signals from various sources after they have been uplinked. For example, actigraphic data from sensors worn on the wrist or sewn into clothing could be combined offline with optical, electrochemical (amperometric measures of glucose and lactic acid), and acoustic/piezoelectric sensors. Many chip-based sensors are currently available, including some measuring oxyhemoglobin, temperature, hemoglobin, hematocrit, and bilirubin. Biological Micro-Electro-Mechanical (BioMEMS) technology has already found applications for sensing viruses, DNA strands, microorganisms, and a variety of molecules. Ambulatory integration of advanced sensor technologies provide remote monitoring capabilities for patients with pulmonary disease, heart failure, and diabetes. Devices in or on the mattress can detect movement, respiration, and heartbeat. Standing waveform generator/detectors sitting at bedside can do likewise. Integrating the signals from multiple sources could provide a much more detailed picture of sleep than we currently have. Smartphones and wristwatchlike devices are currently spearheading this movement. These devices had built in accelerometers and can interface with other transduces using their Wi-Fi and Bluetooth capabilities and then uplink data for processing, summary, and storage (see Ingo Fietze's article, "Sleep Applications to Assess Sleep Quality," in this issue). Smartphones provide a widely extant technologic foundation for developing sleep monitors with minimal additional expense.

It is possible to build such large arrays of data. If data collection devices are noninvasive and automatic (eg, sewn into clothing or incorporated into the bed), cloud computing resources with ample memory could log information from millions of sensors over long periods of time. Thus, changes in these multiple source biometric composites could be correlated with health-related changes both acutely just leading up to illness and chronically over the life span. Now, one might ask, is this polysomnography? The general definition for polysomnography is the simultaneous and continuous monitoring of physiologic activity during sleep. The AASM Standardized Manuel provides specific details.[9] As such, this new integration may not meet strict definitional criteria. Nonetheless, POLY + SOMNO + GRAM, derives

from the combining forms of the Greek "poly" meaning much or many, the Latin "somno" meaning sleep, and the Greek "gram" meaning drawing or something written. Thus, in spirit, the term polysomnography may apply. As with the word itself, polysomnography (recording, methodology, and analysis) will need to redefine itself and evolve least it become a historical footnote.

In its evolved form, what challenges will face polysomnography? Most likely to continue exploring the exact same questions for which it was originally conceived; that is, to provide an objective tool for studying sleep.

REFERENCES

1. Kleitman N. Sleep and wakefulness. Chicago: University of Chicago Press; 1967.
2. Berger H. Über das Elektroenkelphalogramm des Mensen. Arch Pyschiatr Nervenkr 1929;87:527–70.
3. Loomis AL, Harvey N, Hobart GA. Cerebral states during sleep, as studied by human brain potentials. J Exp Psychol 1937;21:127–44.
4. Aserinsky E, Kleitman N. Regularly occurring periods of eye motility, and concomitant phenomena, during sleep. Science 1953;118:273–4.
5. Rechtschaffen A, Kales A. A manual of standardized terminology, techniques and scoring system for sleep stages in human subjects. Washington, DC: U.S. Government Printing Office; 1968. NIH Publication No. 204.
6. Jouvet M, Michel F. Sur les voies nerveuses responsables de l'activité rapide au cours du sommeil physiologique chez le chat (phase paradoxale). CR Soc Biol 1960;154:995–8.
7. Williams RL, Karacan I, editors. Sleep disorders: diagnosis and treatment. New York: John Wiley and Sons; 1979.
8. Guilleminault C, editor. Sleeping and waking disorders: indications and techniques. Menlo Park (CA): Addison-Wesley; 1982.
9. Iber C, Ancoli-Israel S, Chesson A, et al. For the American Academy of Sleep Medicine: the AASM manual for the scoring of sleep and associated events: rules, terminology and technical specifications. Westchester (NY): American Academy of Sleep Medicine; 2007.
10. Chesson AL Jr, Ferber RA, Fry JM, et al. The indications for polysomnography and related procedures. Sleep 1997;20:423–87.
11. Punjabi NM, Welch D, Strohl K. Sleep disorders in regional sleep centers: a national cooperative study. Coleman II Study Investigators. Sleep 2000;23(4):471–80.
12. Huffington post article online. Available at: http://www.huffingtonpost.com/2013/01/03/sleep-centers-highest-number-american-academy-of-sleep-medicine_n_2366719.html. Accessed June 6, 2016.

13. Sackett D. Rules of evidence and clinical recommendation. Can J Cardiol 1993;9:487–9.
14. Kushida CA, Littner MR, Morgenthaler T. Practice parameters for the indications for polysomnography and related procedures: an update for 2005. Sleep 2005;28:499–521.
15. Collop NA, Anderson WM, Boehlecke B, et al. Clinical guidelines for the use of unattended portable monitors in the diagnosis of obstructive sleep apnea in adult patients. J Clin Sleep Med 2007;3(7):737–47.
16. Littner M, Hirshkowitz M, Davila D, et al. Practice parameters for the use of auto-titrating continuous positive airway pressure devices for titrating pressures and treating adult patients with obstructive sleep apnea syndrome. An American Academy of Sleep Medicine report. Sleep 2002;25:143–7.
17. Morgenthaler TI, Aurora RN, Brown T, et al. Standards of Practice Committee of the AASM. Practice parameters for the use of autotitrating continuous positive airway pressure devices for titrating pressures and treating adult patients with obstructive sleep apnea syndrome: an update for 2007. Sleep 2008;31(1): 141–7.
18. EEG arousals: scoring rules and examples: a preliminary report from the Sleep Disorders Atlas Task Force of the American Sleep Disorders Association. Sleep 1992;15:173–84.
19. Terzano MG, Parrino L, Smerieri A, et al. Atlas, rules, and recording technique for scoring of cyclic alternating pattern (CAP) in human sleep. Sleep Med 2002;3:187–99.

Quantifying Leg Movement Activity During Sleep

Raffaele Ferri, MD[a],*, Stephany Fulda, PhD[b]

KEYWORDS

- Periodic leg movements during sleep • Periodic leg movements during wakefulness
- Alternating leg muscle activation • Hypnagogic foot tremor • High-frequency leg movements
- Excessive fragmentary myoclonus

KEY POINTS

- The recording and scoring of limb movement activity during sleep is an essential component in the characterization of periodic leg movements during sleep.
- Currently, 2 sets of similar (but not identical) rules for recording and scoring periodic leg movements during wakefulness and sleep exist.
- Periodic limb movements are the most frequent type of activity during sleep. However, also other, less frequent limb movement activities can be recorded.
- Digital recording of leg muscle electromyography during a nocturnal polysomnography represents the gold standard method.
- Several elements of the current rules lack an empirical foundation and recent data-driven studies are expected to give the basis for new and improved rules.

INTRODUCTION

The recording and scoring of leg movement activity (LMA) during sleep is an essential component in the characterization of sleep and a required component in the assessment of periodic leg movements (PLMs) during sleep (PLMS). Besides characterizing PLMS, there are several other leg movement (LM) patterns, mostly high-frequency, which can be identified during sleep, such as alternating leg muscle activation (ALMA), hypnagogic foot tremor (HFT), or high-frequency LMs (HFLMs).[1]

Currently, 2 sets of similar (but not identical) rules for recording and scoring PLMS and PLMs during wakefulness (PLMW) exist. These were partly informed by algorithms proposed for the automatic detection of LMs in polysomnographic (PSG) recordings [2] and include mathematically defined parameters such as thresholds, intervals, and amplitude.[3,4] First, in 2006 a task force of the International Restless Legs Syndrome Study Group endorsed by the World Association of Sleep Medicine (WASM/IRLSSG)[5] introduced a major revision of the scoring rules, which were then substantially (but not entirely) adopted by the American Academy of Sleep Medicine (AASM) in 2007,[6] and are being periodically updated.[7] Scoring criteria for LMs other than PLMS are specified in the AASM rules.

Funding Sources: Dr R. Ferri, Italian Ministry of Health ("Ricerca Corrente"); Dr S. Fulda, Swiss National Science Foundations (Grant No. 320030_160009).
Conflict of Interest: Nil.

[a] Department of Neurology I.C., Sleep Research Centre, Oasi Institute for Research on Mental Retardation and Brain Aging (IRCCS), Via C. Ruggero, 73, Troina 94018, Italy; [b] Neurocenter of Southern Switzerland, Sleep and Epilepsy Center, Civic Hospital (EOC) of Lugano, Via Tesserete 46, Lugano 6903, Switzerland
* Corresponding author.
E-mail address: rferri@oasi.en.it

Sleep Med Clin 11 (2016) 413–420
http://dx.doi.org/10.1016/j.jsmc.2016.08.005
1556-407X/16/© 2016 Elsevier Inc. All rights reserved.

This article reviews the basic recording methods, scoring rules, and computer-based automatic detection programs for LMA during sleep with a focus on PLMS, the most frequent type of LMA during sleep.

BASIC RECORDING METHODS
Electromyography

Surface electromyography (EMG) is the gold standard for recording leg muscle activity during sleep. It is acquired by means of silver-chloride electrodes attached to the inputs of a differential amplifier to obtain a bipolar derivation. It is usually recommended that interelectrode impedance should be at least less than 10 KΩ (but better <5 KΩ).[5] The skin preparation procedure, before electrode placement, is very important and may include shaving any excess hair, cleaning the skin with alcohol pads, and light abrasion. For a better adhesion of the electrodes, the use of collodion is recommended because it is nonconductive; holds through hair (not only on the scalp), oils, and perspiration; and provides high performance for long-term recordings. However, collodion is highly flammable and produces fumes; thus, appropriate air purifier, fume extractor, or ventilation systems should be used. Finally, a conductive paste for long-term recordings must be used to ensure a good electrical contact between the skin and the electrodes.

Surface EMG electrodes should be placed at 2 to 3 cm apart or one-third of the length of the anterior tibialis muscle, whichever is shorter. Electrodes must be located longitudinally on the muscles, symmetrically around the middle. EMG signals must be obtained from both the right and the left leg, and recording the 2 signals in 1 channel is strongly discouraged. Baseline resting EMG amplitude (ie, in the relaxed muscle) should be ± 2 to 3 μV (4–6 μV peak-to-peak; WASM/IRLSSG)[5] or 10 μV or less (AASM).[7] The WASM/IRLSSG rules recommend that, before the recording, a calibration should be carried out to obtain from the relaxed anterior tibialis muscles a nonrectified signal no greater than ± 5 μV (or 10 μV peak-to-peak, 5 μV for rectified signals) for clinical purposes, and ± 3 μV (or 6 μV peak-to-peak, 3 μV for rectified signals).[5]

EMG signals are produced by the muscle situated under the skin and adipose tissue below the electrodes, which are able to record activity of superficial muscle. Muscle size and amount of adipose tissue significantly influence the amplitude of the surface recorded EMG signal. This is the reason why surface EMG signals are considered semiquantitative and calibration of EMG activity is recommended.[5] The amplitude of surface EMG potentials depends also on the distance between the recording electrodes and can range between less than 20 μV and up to several mV, depending on the factors previously listed.

EMG signals are constituted of superimposed motor unit action potentials produced by several motor units, each with a typical repetition rate of firing of about 7 to 20 Hz. Surface EMG records the sum of this activity and produces a signal with a wide spectrum. Thus, the spectral content of the EMG signal requires high sampling rates that should never be lower than 200 Hz; 400 to 500 Hz are usually recommended.[5,7] Band-pass filtering is usually applied, with typical settings at approximately 10 to 100 Hz and with a notch filter at 50 or 60 Hz, depending on the power line frequency.

Actigraphy

Actigraphy refers to devices whose sensors integrate motion amplitude and speed, and whose output is a signal with magnitude and duration, depending on these motion features. This signal is appropriately amplified, filtered, and digitized to be stored in the device memory, most often in terms of movement counts per epoch. The length of the epoch is of crucial importance and can be fixed at 1 minute or can be chosen by the user (from a fixed list of epoch lengths). Epoch length is very important because, in conjunction with the memory capacity of the device, it determines the maximum recording time. Data are stored essentially in 3 different ways by actigraphs. Some of them allow the user to select the preferred mode, whereas others do not. With the time-above-threshold mode, the amount of time per epoch during which activity exceeds the set threshold is stored. The zero-crossing mode assesses the number of times per epoch that the activity signal produced by the accelerometer crosses a threshold set around zero. Finally, with the proportional-integration (or digital) mode, the area under the curve is stored for each epoch. Some devices allow the simultaneous use of multiple modes. There are no conclusive statements in the literature on which is the most accurate among these modes.

Actigraphy is typically worn at the wrist to monitor rest-activity cycles for several days or weeks; however, for the assessment of LMA, actigraphic monitoring of foot movements or LMs has been proposed.[8,9] When used for the assessment of LMA, sampling rate of the actigraphy must be considerably higher: 10 Hz or more.[5] Because it offers the possibility to record multiple nights in a home environment, it has been proposed as a tool to overcome the problems caused by the relatively large night-to-night within-subject variability reported to occur for PLMS.[10] However, actigraphy alone is unable to discriminate between PLMS and LMs occurring during wakefulness; moreover, arousals or other related events (apnea) cannot be detected.

A recent review and meta-analysis on the use of actigraphy for the measurement of PLMS has demonstrated significant heterogeneity among the few studies available for type of actigraph, position of the sensors on the legs, and methods for counting PLMS.[11] In particular, an important limitation was noted in the inability to reliably combine data from actigraphs placed on both limbs, in most devices.

Thus, currently, actigraphy cannot substitute EMG recording within a nocturnal polysomnography for characterization of LMA during sleep.

Other Methods

Several producers propose piezoelectric sensors for the recording of limb movements during sleep. These sensors, placed around the ankle or around the leg, transduce motion, vibration, and tension into an electrical signal. They are very sensitive and there is no warranty that the signal produced corresponds exclusively to events generated by the limb. There are no convincing validation studies for the use of these sensors and they are not recommended by any guideline. The only advantage that they offer is that they do not need skin preparation; however, this is counterbalanced by a cost higher than that of silver chloride electrodes.

IDENTIFICATION OF LEG MOVEMENTS DURING SLEEP

The basis for the classification and scoring of LMA during sleep is the identification of single LM events. According to current standard rules, their onset is defined as an EMG increase of 8 µV or more above the resting baseline, whereas the offset is marked at the point when the EMG amplitude decreases to less than 2 µV above the resting level and remains below that value for at least 0.5 of a second. An event can contain 1 or more periods with EMG amplitude below the offset level that last less than 0.5 second each. The duration of the event is the time between its onset and offset; it must be at least 0.5 second and no longer than 10 seconds. Currently, all other LMA events not meeting these criteria are discarded and not considered any further, at least for the scoring of PLMS.

SCORING OF LEG MOVEMENTS DURING SLEEP
Periodic Limb Movements

The scoring of PLMS involves several sequential steps. After the identification of individual, monolateral LMs, these are combined to bilateral LMs if they occur near each other. LMs in the vicinity of sleep-disordered breathing events are identified and excluded, and the remaining LMs are classified as periodic or nonperiodic (isolated) based on their occurrence within a series of LMs characterized by their number and the interval between movements. **Fig. 1** shows, as an example, a PSG recording fragment with PLMS in a patient with restless legs syndrome (RLS).

As previously mentioned, there are currently 2 standard set of rules for the scoring of PLMS, the 2006 WASM/IRLSSG rules[5] and the continuously updated AASM rules, with the latest update published in 2016.[7] Although the 2 sets are very similar, even today there remain several critical differences in the rules that are listed in **Table 1**.

One of these differences concerns the rule to combine monolateral LMs to bilateral LMs. The WASM/IRLSSG criteria consider LMs as bilateral if the offset of the first event is less than 0.5 second before the onset of the subsequent

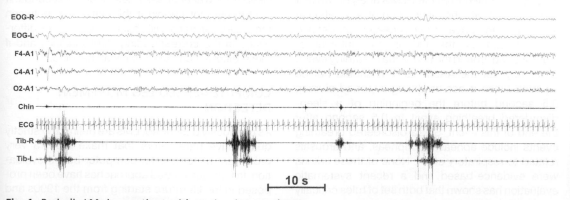

Fig. 1. Periodic LMs in a patient with restless legs syndrome.

Table 1
Critical differences between current scoring rules for periodic leg movements

	WASM/IRLSSG[5]	AASM[7]
Scoring of periodic LMs		
Sleep or Wake	All LMs form PLM series For PLMS, only those during sleep are counted	Only LMs during sleep form PLM series. A PLMS series continues across intermittent wake periods <90 s; in this case, LMs during wake are ignored.
Bilateral LMs	Offset-to-onset <0.5 s	Onset-to-onset <5 s
Respiratory-related LMs (RRLM)	Excluded from PLM series	Excluded from PLM series
RRLM definition	Any LM occurring within ±0.5 s around the ending of an apnea or hypopnea event	Any LM occurring within 0.5 s before the start to 0.5 s after the end of an apnea, hypopnea, respiratory effort–related arousal, or sleep-disordered breathing event

event. In contrast, the AASM rules consider LMs as bilateral if the onset of the first event is less than 5 seconds before the onset of the next event. Because LMs can be between 0.5 second and 10 seconds, the AASM rule also classifies some overlapping LMs as bilateral. None of the 2 sets of rules report a rationale for their choice of the specific criteria for bilateral movements. Despite these differences, a recent study has shown that, in patients with RLS, in the overwhelming majority of events, bilateral LMs are overlapping with each other and are correctly identified by both the current WASM/IRLSSG and AASM rules.[4] Although the 2 set of rules differ considerably in their definition of bilateral LMs, they provided largely corresponding classifications in subjects with RLS and could be considered equivalent in a clinical context.[4]

Both sets of rules exclude LMs that occur in the vicinity of sleep-disordered breathing events (ie, respiratory-related LMs [RRLMs]), from the inclusion into PLMS series and these LMs have to be identified and excluded before determining the PLMS index. For the WASM/IRLSSG rules, a LM must be excluded from the PLMS analysis when it is associated with the resumption of respiration at the end of an apnea or hypopnea event, defined as any part of the LM in the interval of ±0.5 second around the end of the breathing event. Differently, for the AASM, an LM should not be counted when it occurs during a period starting 0.5 second before the beginning of a sleep-disordered breathing event to 0.5 second after the end of this event. Sleep-disordered breathing events include apneas, hypopneas, and arousals related to respiratory effort. None of these criteria were evidence-based and a recent systematic evaluation has shown that both set of rules critically underestimate the number of LMs associated with

respiratory events, which are systematically increased around the end of respiratory events, over a period significantly longer than specified in either set of rules (−2 s to +10.25 s).[12]

Both set of rules agree that, subsequently to combining monolateral LMs and excluding RRLMs, a periodic sequence is defined as a series of 4 or more LMs separated from each other by 5 to 90 seconds. A further crucial point at this step is the question of whether only LMs during sleep or also during wake are part of a PLM series, and how intervening wakefulness affects a possible PLM series. Here, the WASM/IRLSSG rules[5] recommend that all LMs during sleep and wake can form part of a PLM series, and that, for the computation of the PLMS index, only those during sleep are counted. PLMs during wake are counted for the PLMW index. In contrast, the most recent AASM rules[7] state that if the intervening wakefulness is short (<90 s), any LM occurring during wake is ignored and the PLM series continues across this period, provided that the distance between the last LM during sleep before the wakefulness and the first LM during sleep after wakefulness is less than 90 seconds. It is currently not known if this difference between the 2 sets of rules will result in significant differences in the corresponding PLMS indices and if these differences have a clinical meaning.

COMPUTER-BASED LEG MOVEMENT DETECTION

As previously described, LMs are defined by strictly quantitative parameters that make them a very prominent candidate for computer-based evaluation. In fact, automated approaches have been proposed in the literature starting from the 1990s and all of the methods were reported to perform quite well. Kayed and colleagues[13] reported the performance of an undisclosed algorithm applied by a recording system commercially available at that time (1990) and now obsolete, which showed a sensitivity of 94% and a specificity of 85%. Further algorithms were published by Tauchmann and Pollmächer[14] in 1996; Roessen and colleagues[15] in 1998; and Wetter and colleagues,[16] and Pittman and colleagues,[17] in 2004.

In 2005, Ferri and colleagues[2] described a detection of LMs performed by using 2 thresholds:

1 for the starting point and another to detect the end point of each LM. Values of sensitivity and specificity of 90% or more were found in all recordings and sensitivity and false-positive rates were used to set up amplitude cutoff values for the 2 thresholds. These values were subsequently adopted by both the current sets of internationally accepted criteria to detect PLMS.

There has been a recent renewed interest in LM or PLM detectors (**Table 2**). Moore and colleagues[18] have described another method

Table 2
Overview of computer-based leg movement detection algorithms

Study	Sample	Key Features of the Algorithm	Main Results
Kayed et al,[13] 1990	10 recordings of subjects with PLMS	Not described in detail	PLM event count Sensitivity 94% Specificity 85%
Tauchmann & Pollmächer,[14] 1996	10 recordings of 5 subjects with RLS	Threshold and bridge criteria	LM detection Sensitivity 93% Specificity 89%–92%
Roessen et al,[15] 1998	30 recordings of subjects with PLMD	Amplitude thresholding after various filter operations	No significant differences in %PLM/TIB and LMI/TIB; LMI/TST higher with the automatic scoring
Wetter et al,[16] 2004	10 recordings of subjects with RLS	Pattern recognition based on burst density, amplitude, and duration	LM detection Sensitivity 94%
Pittman et al,[17] 2004	31 recordings of subjects with various sleep disorders	Adaptive segmentation based on relative energy of time-frequency features	PLM detection Agreement 92%–93%
Ferri et al,[2] 2005	Recordings of 15 RLS/PLMS and 15 control subjects	Amplitude thresholding after filtering and rectifying	LM detection Sensitivity $\geq$90% Specificity $\geq$90%
Moore et al,[18] 2014	Recordings of 78 subjects with various sleep disorders	Adaptive noise cancellation and noise adjusted threshold detections	PLM detection Sensitivity 73%–77% Specificity 99%–100%
Huang et al,[19] 2015	Recordings of 15 RLS and 9 control subjects	Amplitude thresholding after filtering	PLM detection Sensitivity 96% Specificity 92%
Alverez-Estevez,[20] 2016	70 recordings of subjects with various sleep disorders	Various filter operations and dynamic baseline determination	PLM detection Average sensitivity 82% specificity 100%
Shokrollahi et al,[21] 2016	65 subjects with stroke, TIA, or other diagnoses	Kernel sparse representation of K-nonnegative matrix factorization of the signal time-frequency matrices	PLM index $\geq$30 Overall accuracy 97%

Abbreviations: LMI, leg movement index; PLM, periodic leg movements; TIA, transient ischemic attack; TIB, time in bed; TST, total sleep time.

characterized by adaptive noise canceling of cardiac artifacts and noise-floor adjustable detection thresholds with promising performance. They have made the code public for use in personalized applications and modification. A further, interesting and promising algorithm has been published by Huang and colleagues,[19] who have made a MATLAB script publicly available and have underlined the need for a good reference human scoring when assessing the performance of automatic systems that might be adjusted better if an accurate and expert scoring is used. Alvarez-Estevez[20] proposed a detection method based on various filter operations and the determination of an adjusted baseline. Finally, Shokrollahi and colleagues[21] have proposed an algorithm involving time frequency matrices, K-nonnegative matrix factorization, and kernel sparse representation.

All these studies seem to indicate that PLMS can be detected reliably by means of computer-based automatic approaches. All of these approaches, however, suffer from the unknown precision of the human gold standard because all algorithms have been validated against a limited number of human scorers with varying degrees of experience and always within a single sleep center. It is currently unknown what the inter-center agreement of manual LM scorings is, which will be a limiting factor for any validation of automatic detection algorithms.

OTHER LEG MOTOR ACTIVITIES DURING SLEEP

This section includes other phenomena of small motor activations of the feet (and legs) occurring at sleep onset, usually in trains, with short lasting bilateral alternating or unilateral (agonist or antagonist) activations. According to current knowledge they are all considered benign movement phenomena.

Alternating Leg Muscle Activation

The term ALMA during sleep indicates a quickly alternating pattern of anterior tibialis activations occurring at a frequency from 0.5 Hz to 3 Hz. The usual duration of a single leg muscle activation within an ALMA pattern is 100 to 500 milliseconds, and at least 4 alternating activations are needed to form an ALMA series. The phenomenon was reported to occur in all sleep stages but particularly during arousals.[22,23] It is not clear yet if ALMA represents the PSG manifestation of a separate nosologic entity or if it belongs to the wide spectrum of nocturnal motor activities of RLS. **Fig. 2** shows, as an example, 2 consecutive ALMA episodes during sleep in a patient.[23]

Hypnagogic Foot Tremor

HFT, described later by others[24] but first in 1988 by Broughton,[25] is a clinical condition that has several similarities to ALMA: subjects exhibit repetitive foot movements occurring at the transition between wake and sleep or during light sleep. PSG recordings show the presence of recurrent EMG potentials (at least 4) or foot movements typically at 1 to 2 Hz (range 0.3–4 Hz) in 1 or both feet. The EMG bursts are longer than those of myoclonus (250–1000 ms), and are organized in trains of variable length.

High-Frequency Leg Movements

The term HFLM was recently proposed for a similar phenomenon.[26] HFLM was defined as 4 or more discrete LMs occurring at a frequency of 0.3 to 4 Hz, unilaterally, but sometimes with a bilateral pattern. Two-thirds of the HFLM are observed during waking and approximately one-third during sleep. However, the criteria to score this

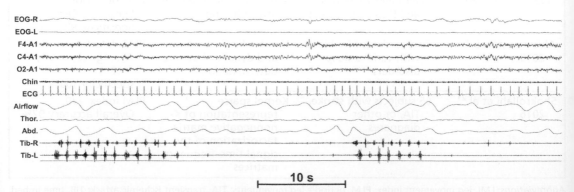

Fig. 2. Two consecutive ALMA episodes during sleep in a patient reported by Cosentino and colleagues.[23]

phenomenon have not been established, and additional studies and reports are needed to define their eventual relationship with RLS and their clinical relevance.

Excessive Fragmentary Myoclonus

Excessive fragmentary myoclonus (EFM) is characterized by an abundance (>20 minutes) of very short EMG bursts, which are usually less than 150 milliseconds. EFM is a very common phenomenon, even in healthy sleepers.[27]

SUMMARY

The recording and scoring of LMA during sleep is well established and has been standardized according to international guidelines. Digital recording of leg muscle EMG during a nocturnal polysomnography represents the gold standard. At the same time, scoring criteria are the results of a dynamic process that reflects the progress in clinical sleep medicine and research, and several elements of the current rules lack an empirical foundation. It is, therefore, expected that scoring rules will undergo further changes as new evidence emerges.

REFERENCES

1. American Academy of Sleep Medicine. International classification of sleep disorders. 3rd edition. Darien (IL): American Academy of Sleep Medicine; 2014.
2. Ferri R, Zucconi M, Manconi M, et al. Computer-assisted detection of nocturnal leg motor activity in patients with restless legs syndrome and periodic leg movements during sleep. Sleep 2005;28(8):998–1004.
3. Ferri R, Rundo F, Zucconi M, et al. An evidence-based analysis of the association between periodic leg movements during sleep and arousals in restless legs syndrome. Sleep 2015;38(6):919–24.
4. Ferri R, Manconi M, Rundo F, et al. A data-driven analysis of the rules defining bilateral leg movements during sleep. Sleep 2016;39:413–21.
5. Zucconi M, Ferri R, Allen R, et al. The official World Association of Sleep Medicine (WASM) standards for recording and scoring periodic leg movements in sleep (PLMS) and wakefulness (PLMW) developed in collaboration with a task force from the International Restless Legs Syndrome Study Group (IRLSSG). Sleep Med 2006;7(2):175–83.
6. Iber C, Ancoli-Israel S, Chesson AL, et al. The AASM manual for the scoring of sleep and associated events: rules, terminology, and technical specifications. 1st edition. Westchester (IL): American Academy of Sleep Medicine; 2007.
7. Berry RB, Brooks R, Gamaldo CE, et al. The AASM manual for the scoring of sleep and associated events: rules, terminology and technical specifications, Ver. 2.3. Darien (IL): American Academy of Sleep Medicine; 2016.
8. Allen RP. Improving RLS diagnosis and severity assessment: polysomnography, actigraphy and RLS-sleep log. Sleep Med 2007;8(Suppl 2):S13–8.
9. Sforza E, Zamagni M, Petiav C, et al. Actigraphy and leg movements during sleep: a validation study. J Clin Neurophysiol 1999;16(2):154–60.
10. Trotti LM, Bliwise DL, Greer SA, et al. Correlates of PLMs variability over multiple nights and impact upon RLS diagnosis. Sleep Med 2009;10(6):668–71.
11. Plante DT. Leg actigraphy to quantify periodic limb movements of sleep: a systematic review and meta-analysis. Sleep Med Rev 2014;18(5):425–34.
12. Manconi M, Zavalko I, Fanfulla F, et al. An evidence-based recommendation for a new definition of respiratory-related leg movements. Sleep 2015; 38(2):295–304.
13. Kayed K, Roberts S, Davies WL. Computer detection and analysis of periodic movements in sleep. Sleep 1990;13(3):253–61.
14. Tauchmann N, Pollmächer T. Automatic detection of periodic leg movements (PLM). J Sleep Res 1996; 5(4):273–5.
15. Roessen M, Thijssen M, Kemp B. Semi-automatic detection of leg movements: program features and scoring results. In: Beersma DGM, van Bemmel AL, Folgering H, et al, editors. Sleep-wake research in The Netherlands, vol. 9. Leiden (The Netherlands): Dutch Society for Sleep-Wake Research; 1998. p. 101–5.
16. Wetter TC, Dirlich G, Streit J, et al. An automatic method for scoring leg movements in polygraphic sleep recordings and its validity in comparison to visual scoring. Sleep 2004;27(2):324–8.
17. Pittman SD, MacDonald MM, Fogel RB, et al. Assessment of automated scoring of polysomnographic recordings in a population with suspected sleep-disordered breathing. Sleep 2004;27(7): 1394–403.
18. Moore H, Leary E, Lee SY, et al. Design and validation of a periodic leg movement detector. PLoS One 2014;9(12):e114565.
19. Huang AS, Skeba P, Yang MS, et al. MATPLM1, A MATLAB script for scoring of periodic limb movements: preliminary validation with visual scoring. Sleep Med 2015;16(12):1541–9.
20. Alvarez-Estevez D. A new automatic method for the detection of limb movements and the analysis of their periodicity. Biomed Sign Process Control 2016;26:117–25.
21. Shokrollahi M, Krishnan S, Dopsa DD, et al. Nonnegative matrix factorization and sparse representation for the automated detection of periodic limb movements in sleep. Med Biol Eng Comput 2016. [Epub ahead of print].
22. Chervin RD, Consens FB, Kutluay E. Alternating leg muscle activation during sleep and arousals: a new

sleep-related motor phenomenon? Mov Disord 2003;18(5):551–9.

23. Cosentino FI, Iero I, Lanuzza B, et al. The neurophysiology of the alternating leg muscle activation (ALMA) during sleep: study of one patient before and after treatment with pramipexole. Sleep Med 2006;7(1):63–71.

24. Wichniak A, Tracik F, Geisler P, et al. Rhythmic feet movements while falling asleep. Mov Disord 2001; 16(6):1164–70.

25. Broughton R. Pathological fragmentary myoclonus, intensified hypnic jerks and hypnagogic foot tremor:

three unusual sleep-related movement disorders. In: Koella WP, Obal F, Schultz H, et al, editors. Sleep 86. Suttgart (Germany): Gustav Fischer Verlag; 1988. p. 240–2.

26. Yang C, Winkelman JW. Clinical and polysomnographic characteristics of high frequency leg movements. J Clin Sleep Med 2010;6(5):431–8.

27. Frauscher B, Kunz A, Brandauer E, et al. Fragmentary myoclonus in sleep revisited: a polysomnographic study in 62 patients. Sleep Med 2011; 12(4):410–5.

Quantifying Airflow Limitation and Snoring During Sleep

Erna Sif Arnardottir, PhD[a,b,*], Thorarinn Gislason, PhD, MD[a,b]

KEYWORDS

- Flow limitation • Respiratory effort • Snore • Esophageal pressure • Pneumotachography

KEY POINTS

- This article aids readers to understand the advantages and limitations of current techniques to assess obstructive breathing in the absence of classical obstructive sleep apnea.
- Current techniques to measure obstructive breathing, by measuring flow limitation, respiratory effort, and snoring, are all nonstandardized making it difficult to assess their clinical consequences.
- Standardization of measurements for obstructive breathing is crucial for understanding its true pathophysiologic significance independent of downstream effects, such as oxygen desaturations and arousals.

INTRODUCTION: NATURE OF THE PROBLEM

Breathing during sleep through an airway dimension that is too small for the ventilatory need of a given person is associated with different levels of upper airway obstruction. Such obstructive breathing cannot be measured directly but is reflected in flow limitation (flattening of the inspiratory flow waveform), increased respiratory effort, and/or snoring. More severe airway obstruction causes decreased airflow in an oscillatory manner (hypopneas) and breathing cessations (apneas). In the continuum of sleep-disordered breathing (SDB) from mild airway obstruction to moderate/severe obstructive sleep apnea (OSA), diagnosis is based almost solely on the number of apneas and hypopneas, by assessing the apnea-hypopnea index (AHI) per hour. The AHI successfully identifies subjects with the most severe obstructive breathing but not the milder forms of SDB. The pathophysiologic consequences of OSA have, however, been found to be more closely related to the oxygen desaturation index than the AHI itself.[1–4] Similarly, subjects with upper airway resistance syndrome (UARS) are characterized by obstructive breathing events only if the events are associated with arousals,[5] otherwise the obstructive breathing is not assessed. Further work is needed to characterize the pathophysiology and adverse effects of different degrees of obstructive breathing independently from downstream events, such as arousals and oxygen desaturations. This may be especially important in populations where the AHI is relatively low, such as in younger adults (<40 years),[6] children,[7] and in pregnancy[8–10] where there are indications of possible adverse effects of obstructive breathing in the absence of traditional apneas and hypopneas.

Quantifying obstructive breathing is, however, of limited clinical use because there is no standardization of the actual techniques. This limits the application of these measurements, and different sleep laboratories use different sensors and

Disclosure: E.S. Arnardottir is a part-time consultant for Nox Medical and has received an honorarium from Weinmann. T. Gislason holds 0.76% of shares in Nox Medical and has received lecture fees from Nox Medical.
[a] Department of Respiratory Medicine and Sleep, Landspitali – The National University Hospital of Iceland, Fossvogur (E7), Reykjavik 108, Iceland; [b] Faculty of Medicine, University of Iceland, Reykjavik, Iceland
* Corresponding author. Department of Respiratory Medicine and Sleep, Landspitali – The National University Hospital of Iceland, Fossvogur (E7), Reykjavik 108, Iceland.
E-mail address: ernasif@landspitali.is

different rules for scoring of events for their assessment.[11] This makes it difficult to assess the clinical relevance of these measurements and to set standards for clinical guidelines. In the following sections, the characteristics of the current available techniques for assessing obstructive breathing in clinical sleep studies are summarized. This article helps readers understand the advantages and limitations of current techniques.

TECHNIQUE FOR ASSESSMENT OF OBSTRUCTIVE BREATHING DURING SLEEP

The number of techniques available to assess obstructive breathing is high. This review focuses on the invasive methods typically considered gold standard for assessing obstructive breathing: pneumotachography for measuring flow, esophageal manometry for measuring respiratory effort, and noninvasive methods that are used to measure obstructive breathing in clinical sleep studies (**Figs. 1** and **2**). **Table 1** shows a summary of available techniques to measure flow limitation, respiratory effort, and snoring.

In the early days of clinical sleep studies, strain gauges and piezoelectric thoracoabdominal belts were used to assess respiratory effort but both are currently considered obsolete techniques and therefore not discussed further.[11] Other

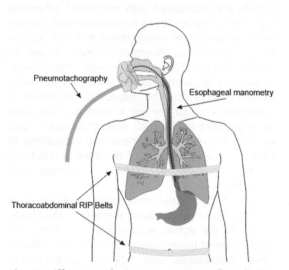

Fig. 1. Different techniques to measure flow limitation and respiratory effort. Quantitative flow is measured by an oronasal mask via pneumotachography. Flow can also be measured qualitatively via the nasal cannula (shown in **Fig. 2**). Quantitative respiratory effort is measured via a catheter placed in the esophagus measuring esophageal pressure. Respiratory effort is also measured indirectly via respiratory inspiratory plethysmography (RIP) belts placed on the thorax and abdomen.

sensors that measure airflow directly but qualitatively, such as a thermistor[12] and end-tidal capnography,[13] which are not sensitive to flow limitation are also not covered by this review. Also, other invasive methods, aside from pneumotachography and esophageal manometry, which are not considered the gold standard approach are not included in this review. The relative invasiveness of these methods makes it unlikely that they will be included in future clinical sleep studies where the technical development during recent years has favored simpler rather than more complex and invasive methods. For example, now patients referred for sleep apnea testing may have their studies performed as a home type 3 sleep study in many countries instead of an in-laboratory polysomnography (PSG).[11,14] Surrogate markers of obstructive breathing during sleep, such as pulse transit time, which do not attempt to actually measure the obstructive breathing itself are also outside the scope of this review. The clinical usefulness of many of these surrogate markers is currently limited, as is summarized in a review by Vanderbussche and colleagues.[15] Assessment of patient populations with ventilatory center impairment is also outside the scope of this review.

INDICATIONS AND CONTRAINDICATIONS

Both available quantitative measurements, pneumotachography for flow and esophageal manometry for respiratory effort, are cumbersome and uncomfortable for the patient. Nasal cannulas and respiratory inductance plethysmography (RIP) belts are typically included in PSG and type 3 sleep studies and both sensors are generally well accepted even though some children have difficulty tolerating the cannula for the whole night. The microphone is often included in in-laboratory studies and in some home sleep studies. The piezoelectric sensor is not a part of the standard PSG and variably included in studies[11] but is well tolerated.

Pneumotachography studies need to be performed as attended in-laboratory studies where subjects are monitored throughout the night. Side effects may include claustrophobia and noncompliance in a similar manner as is seen with positive airway pressure (PAP) studies.[16] Subjects can be sent home with the esophageal manometry but such studies are usually performed in the sleep laboratory where movements, inadvertent removals of the catheter, and artifacts can be addressed during the study. The adverse effects of esophageal manometry during sleep on adults are debated in the literature[17–19] but

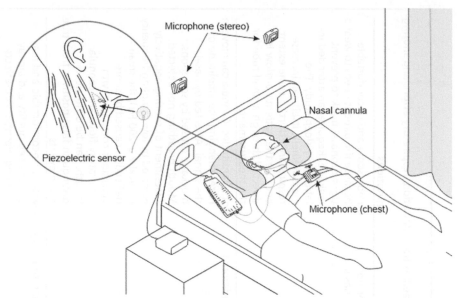

Fig. 2. A comparison of different techniques to measure snoring: cannula measuring vibrations in nares, piezo-electric sensor measuring vibrations on the neck, and microphone measuring loudness on patient chest and on wall in stereo. (*Adapted from* Arnardottir ES, Isleifsson B, Agustsson JS, et al. How to measure snoring? A comparison of the microphone, cannula and piezoelectric sensor. J Sleep Res 2016;25:159.)

most likely the measurements are associated with disturbed sleep, at least in sensitive subjects. These measurements are especially difficult in pediatric studies. Chervin and colleagues[20] found that many families declined participation in a research study using esophageal manometry, and the success rate for a full night study in enrolled subjects was only 61% because of pain, crying at insertion, vomiting, and unintentionally removing the catheter during sleep. Other sensitive groups, such as pregnant women, the elderly, and those with many comorbidities aside from suspected OSA, may find it difficult to participate in such invasive studies.

Potential Complications

Pneumotachography
Special care should be taken when assessing vulnerable populations with limited respiratory drive because the procedure itself may potentially increase respiratory effort to some extent.

Esophageal manometry
If any of the following but highly unlikely scenarios occurs, the catheter should be removed and a doctor notified[21]:

- Excessive coughing that continues for some minutes. May indicate wrong placement of catheter (in trachea).
- Moderate or severe bleeding from the nose or mouth. Minor bleeding caused by bruising of

the mucosa in the nose can occasionally occur.
- Excessive patient anxiety, shortness of breath, or fainting.

No known complications are found for the other sensors discussed here.

REPORTING AND CLINICAL IMPLICATIONS

The technical specifications of the current American Academy of Sleep Medicine manual (2016, version 2.3) recommend that respiratory effort is monitored with esophageal manometry or dual thoracoabdominal RIP belts.[14] However, no further specifications are made for how to score respiratory effort using these methods (see example of tracings in **Fig. 3**). For the scoring of respiratory effort–related arousals (RERAs), the classification of a respiratory effort is a "sequence of ≥ 2 breaths (or duration of two breaths during baseline breathing) when the breathing sequence is characterized by increased respiratory effort, flattening of the inspiratory portion of the nasal pressure (diagnostic study) or PAP device flow (titration study) waveform, snoring, or an elevation in the end-tidal P_{CO_2} leading to arousal from sleep when the sequence of breaths do not meet criteria for an apnea or hypopnea."[14] Again, the definition of increased respiratory effort and flow limitation (referred to as flattening of the inspiratory portion of the nasal pressure) remains vague. Examples

Table 1
The characteristics of different techniques to measure obstructive breathing during sleep, characterized as flow limitation, respiratory effort, and snoring

Sensor	Description of Measurement	Pros	Limitations
Pneumotachography[57–61]	A tight-fitting face mask that measures oronasal inspiratory and expiratory airflow in milliliters (measurement of pressure drop across a linear resistance). The shape of the inspiratory flow curve is used as a measurement of flow limitation.	The reference standard for flow. Quantitative. Measures nasal and mouth breathing.	Cumbersome and uncomfortable because the patient needs to wear a tight oronasal mask to prevent leakage. Requires an attended in-laboratory sleep study. The measurement itself can increase respiratory effort to some extent because the patient's airflow is directed through a small tube for the measurement.
Nasal cannula[22,59,62–66]	Measures air pressure changes at the nares. Included in most clinical sleep studies. The shape of the inspiratory flow curve is used as an indication of flow limitation.	Noninvasive. A part of traditional clinical sleep studies.	Not quantitative. Cannula can move in nares changing the amplitude of the signal. Affected by nasal blockage caused by secretions. Mouth breathing not detected. Assessment of snoring negatively affected by low sampling frequency (typically 0–200 Hz), the small deflection caused by snore vibrations compared with respiratory flow, and cannula length. Can be difficult to distinguish false positives from true snore events.
Esophageal manometry[20,21,67]	Measure pressure in the esophagus, reflecting intrathoracic pressure.	The reference standard for respiratory effort.	Invasive. Uncomfortable and may affect sleep quality and airway opening. Possible side-effects include coughing, gagging, and vomiting. Not included in most routine sleep studies.

Respiratory inductance plethysmography belts[68-70]	Measures thoracoabdominal volume changes. The sum is an indirect measure of lung volume.	Noninvasive. A part of traditional clinical sleep studies.	Not quantitative. An indirect measurement of flow and respiratory effort (by examining paradoxic thoracoabdominal movements). The signal is affected by the position of the subject (eg, sitting, supine) and the belts can move on the patient during the night.
Air-coupled microphone[22,71,72]	Sound measurement for snoring.	Quantitative. Noninvasive. Included in many clinical sleep studies.	Nonstandardized location of microphone (eg, on wall, above patient, forehead, or chest). Ambient noise also recorded. Sound recording needs to be reviewed for false positives.
Piezoelectric sensors[22,73]	Vibration at skin level, usually on neck for snoring.	Noninvasive.	Not quantitative. Does not pick up all snore events. Assessment of snoring affected by low sampling frequency (typically 0–200 Hz). Can be difficult to distinguish false positives from true snore events.

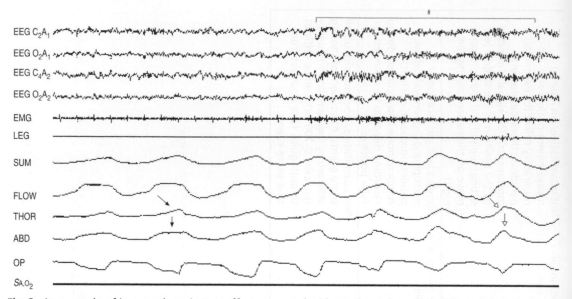

Fig. 3. An example of increased respiratory effort measured with esophageal pressure (OP) and dual thoracoabdominal RIP belts (*black arrows*) compared with normal RIP belts and esophageal pressure (*white arrows*) after an arousal. (*Reproduced from* Masa JF, Corral J, Martín MJ, et al. Assessment of thoracoabdominal bands to detect respiratory effort-related arousal. Eur Respir J 2003;22:663; with permission of the European Respiratory Society.)

of flow-limited breaths are found in **Fig. 4**. Differentiation of apneas by scoring them as obstructive, mixed, or central events does rely on measurements of inspiratory effort during the period of absent airflow without further explanations to how to score absent versus continued inspiratory effort. Similarly, the technical specifications for measuring snoring state that snoring can be assessed with an acoustic sensor (eg, microphone), a piezoelectric sensor, or nasal pressure transducer (cannula) without further specification how to score snore events from these signals because limited comparison has been performed for these sensors.[22] We performed a study comparing these three sensors[22]; an example of snore tracings from that study is shown in **Fig. 5** and further discussed in **Table 2**. In children, the definition of flow limitation, respiratory effort, and snoring is also vague and the scoring of RERAs is optional.[5,14] For further technical details, see **Table 2**. For a detailed technical protocol for esophageal manometry, see Kushida and colleagues.[21] Independent of method used, manual scoring of events is needed, which is time consuming for breath-to-breath analyses.

Because of the technical limitations and lack of standardization, breathing abnormalities caused by airway obstruction during sleep are not based on different degrees of obstruction but rather on possible consequences, such as arousals. Palombini and colleagues[23] studied more than 1000 adults in a general population sample with no sleep complaints and found that flow limitation of 30% (based on a shape criteria) could be used as the upper bound for normal breathing during sleep. Further studies of this kind are needed.

UARS, first described by Guilleminault and colleagues[24] in 1993, is included in the diagnosis of OSA for adults in the International Classification of Sleep Disorders, third edition, and considered to share the same pathophysiology.[5] UARS is characterized as a variant of OSA where obstructive events lead to an arousal rather than oxygen desaturation.[5] The event scoring therefore includes conventional scoring of obstructive or mixed apneas, hypopneas and optionally scoring RERAs.[5,14] When RERAs are scored, the resulting event index is called respiratory disturbance index (RDI) instead of the traditional AHI.[14] The diagnostic criteria for UARS rather than OSA per se is therefore either an RDI greater than or equal to 5 events per hour with symptoms or patient history or greater than or equal to 15 events per hour with no symptoms where the AHI is less than 5 or 15 per hour, respectively.[5] If home sleep apnea testing is performed (type 3 study), RERAs and hypopneas related to arousals cannot be assessed and therefore if UARS is suspected, a PSG needs to be performed.

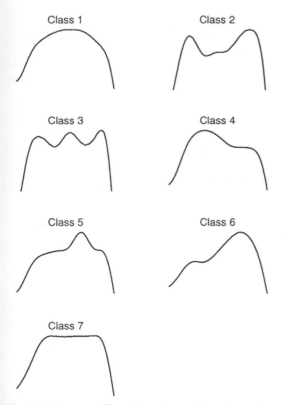

Class 1   Class 2

Class 3   Class 4

Class 5   Class 6

Class 7

Fig. 4. The seven different inspiratory flow shape classes described. Class 1 represents normal inspiration but the other waveforms are interpreted as flow limitation (with the possible exception of class 4). These flow shapes can be measured by pneumotachography or nasal cannula. (*Reprinted from* Aittokallio T, Saaresranta T, Polo-Kantola P, et al. Analysis of inspiratory flow shapes in patients with partial upper-airway obstruction during sleep. Chest 2001;119:39; with permission from Elsevier.)

The optional scoring of RERAs in clinical sleep studies greatly affects the total number of respiratory events scored (RDI vs AHI). This further adds to the discrepancies that already exist when sleep laboratories are using different scoring rules and sensors for classification of OSA events (see further in Ref.[11]). This can cause large differences in the scored AHI.[25,26] Also, the agreement for the scoring of RERA events is probably low (no papers, however, were found on a PubMed search for RERA scoring agreement) because the agreement for hypopnea scoring becomes progressively worse as the definitions become less strict (moving from 4% oxygen desaturation index, to 3% or arousals or $\geq$50% drop in flow signal[25]). Hypopnea scoring agreement is also affected by the flow sensor used and is worse for raw nasal pressure and RIP belt scoring than for transformed nasal pressure.[27] Scorer agreement for scoring

arousals is very low, which also impacts RERA scoring.[25,28]

CLINICAL OUTCOMES

Previous research has shown that obstructive breathing without apneas or hypopneas in adults may be related to increased sleep instability as assessed by cyclic alternating pattern,[29] increased sleepiness,[30,31] worse work performance,[32] morning headaches,[33] gastroesophageal reflux,[34,35] local nerve lesions,[36,37] increased blood pressure,[38] and even atherosclerosis of the carotid artery.[39] In children, a history of habitual snoring has been shown to be associated with similar adverse neurocognitive[40] and behavioral[41,42] deficits as in children with OSA. In pregnancy, SDB may be related to negative outcomes for the mother and fetus.[10] Future studies with more standardized measurements focusing not only on the AHI or arousal-related events but also the independent effects of obstructive breathing per se are needed.

It is also important to note that the current diagnostic criteria for OSA,[14,43,44] based on sleep study results alone without any symptoms (when AHI $\geq$15), may be inflating the true prevalence of OSA and causing overdiagnosis and treatment.[45,46] The AHI rises significantly with age.[6,47] Despite the increase in AHI seen in the elderly, the relationship with mortality rate[48,49] and comorbidities, such as hypertension,[50,51] decreases significantly. The increase in AHI in the elderly is also not accompanied by an increase in snoring, which peaks in middle age.[52] Finally, the AHI is not well associated with classical OSA symptoms, such as subjective sleepiness, fatigue, quality of life, and objective vigilance.[30,53] Therefore the question arises whether other indicators of SDB reflecting different degrees of obstructive breathing and respiratory effort could be more appropriate to assess disease severity than the AHI alone.

CURRENT CONTROVERSIES/FUTURE CONSIDERATIONS

Sleep studies using esophageal manometry, pneumotachography, and other cumbersome and invasive measurement techniques will always be relatively few and have low numbers because of the nature of such monitoring. We believe that there is a need for reliable noninvasive methods that are validated against these gold-standard methods in smaller cohorts. Then these noninvasive methods can be applied to much larger epidemiologic and clinical cohorts assessing the clinical

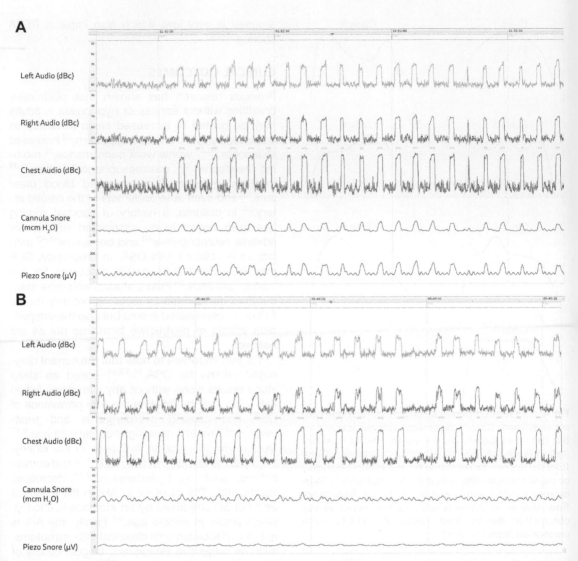

Fig. 5. Examples of true snore events, as measured by the audio (left audio and right audio on wall and chest audio), the nasal cannula, and piezoelectric sensor. (*A*) Snore picked up by all three sensors. (*B*) Snore picked up only by audio, not nasal cannula and piezoelectric sensor, except last two events. The decibel level is lower for the wall audio than the chest audio because the microphones are located further away from the snore source. Both panels are 2 minutes, and signals are shown in the same amplitude in both panels. Manually scored snore events are shown above the tracing on the chest audio channel.

significance of obstructive breathing as reflected in different parameters of flow limitation, respiratory effort, and snoring. These studies need to be cross-sectional and longitudinal and reflect the variety of subjects assessed, from healthy to severely sick and in different populations; children, middle-aged, elderly subjects, and pregnant women because different indices (or a combination of indices) may apply to indicate disease risk for these groups. Also, adults are not a homogenous group; patients with different comorbidities affecting respiration need to be assessed

specifically. For example, at least 1% of the adult population has coexisting chronic obstructive pulmonary disease and OSA, termed the overlap syndrome,[54] and obesity affects the response to SDB.[4,55,56]

Preferably such methods could use information from some of the sensors currently used in clinical sleep studies or could be easily added to such studies. Finding the best way to measure obstructive breathing noninvasively during sleep and knowing the clinical significance of the analysis would enable clinical decision-makers to

Table 2
The signal manipulation, scoring criteria, and available technical validation of the various measurement techniques for obstructive breathing

Sensor Used	Signal Manipulation	Scoring Criteria	Technical Validation
Pneumotachography[14,23,63,64,74–78]	Airflow sampling rate: Typically 0–200 Hz with a high-frequency filter of 100 Hz (excessive filtering may compromise accurate visualization). Calibration needed for each measurement. Increased reliability with heating.	Flow limitation: No uniform criteria. Typically used criteria include: Shape criteria Flattening or oscillations of the inspiratory flow curve. Sometimes classified into 7 subtypes, see **Fig. 4.** Amplitude criteria Decreased airflow $\geq$10 s with a flattened appearance that does not meet criteria for hypopnea.	Reference technique for flow. Shape analysis (both pneumotachography and nasal cannula) has high accuracy for detecting moderate to severe flow limitation characterized as a decrease in esophageal pressure without a corresponding increase in flow rate. Shape analysis, however, does not detect breaths with a high but fixed resistance throughout the inspiration.
Nasal cannula.[14,22,23,59,65,79–81]	Airflow sampling rate: See for pneumotachography. Snoring: 10–100 Hz range to remove the respiratory flow part of the signal. A higher resolution may improve the snore signal.	Flow limitation: See for pneumotachography. Snoring: No uniform criteria. Has been described as in synchrony with breathing and protuberant from background.	Flow limitation: More accurate assessment of flow limitations when signal is square root transformed. Snoring: Missed out on a significant number of true snore events. Performed well in automatic analysis trained on a small set of audio snore data but no scoring rules were included for manual review of the data.
Esophageal manometry[14,15,21,82]	Sampling rate typically 100 Hz. Measured in cm H_2O. Calibration needed for each measurement. Oscillations more reliable than specific nadir levels.	No uniform criteria. Typically used criteria include a crescendo pattern lasting >10 s followed by an abrupt return to baseline. Nadir levels sometimes marked (eg, −10 or −12 cm H_2O). Sometimes events only scored when followed by an arousal. Continuous high effort scored in some studies without crescendo pattern.	Reference technique of respiratory effort.

(continued on next page)

Table 2
(continued)

Sensor Used	Signal Manipulation	Scoring Criteria	Technical Validation
RIP belts[15,69,78,83,84]	Sampling rate typically 100 Hz. Time derivative of RIP sum used to approximate flow. More accurate flow assessment when calibrated.	No uniform criteria. Generally described as paradoxic thoracoabdominal movements. Has also been described as a decrease in thoracoabdominal movements and alteration of the inspiratory shape followed by normalization.	Performed well when assessing events with arousals and/or desaturations. Less accurate when assessed by RIP alone. Shape analysis has less accuracy for detecting flow limitation than the pneumotachography and nasal cannula.
Air-coupled microphone[14,22,85–87]	Sampling rate >4000 kHz recommended. >1 kHz needed to capture the peak of the signal (higher than the recommended AASM sampling rate). Decibel calibration recommended for comparison between studies. dB(A) weighting often performed but dB(C) weighting may be more appropriate.	No uniform criteria. Has been described as in synchrony with breathing and protuberant from background, sometimes with an audible oscillatory component or decibel threshold.	Performed well compared with the cannula and piezoelectric sensor. Performed better when placed on patient than when on wall (further away from snore source).
Piezoelectric sensor[14,22,73,85]	Sampling rate typically 0–200 Hz with filter settings recommended by AASM: 0–100 Hz. A higher resolution may improve the signal.	No uniform criteria. Has been described as In synchrony with breathing and protuberant from background.	Missed out on a significant number of true snore events. Performed well in automatic analysis trained on a small set of audio snore data but no scoring rules for manual overview.

Abbreviation: AASM, American Academy of Sleep Medicine.

decide the optimal treatment on a much more objective ground than currently available. This would be a tremendous help in the huge gray zone between severe OSA and normal breathing.

Subjects who do not have the minimum number of apneas and hypopneas to fulfill criteria for OSA but are symptomatic should currently undergo PSG where obstructive breathing and arousals are assessed by some of the techniques discussed here. Standardized techniques for measuring the degree of obstructive breathing in a given person and its possible physiologic and clinical consequences without assessing only events leading to arousals and/or oxygen desaturations are however, needed.

REFERENCES

1. Dean DA, Wang R, Jacobs DR, et al. A systematic assessment of the association of polysomnographic indices with blood pressure: the Multi-Ethnic Study of Atherosclerosis (MESA). Sleep 2015;38:587–96.

2. Punjabi NM, Newman AB, Young TB, et al. Sleep-disordered breathing and cardiovascular disease: an outcome-based definition of hypopneas. Am J Respir Crit Care Med 2008;177:1150–5.

3. Tkacova R, McNicholas WT, Javorsky M, et al, European Sleep Apnoea Database Study Collaborators. Nocturnal intermittent hypoxia predicts prevalent hypertension in the European Sleep Apnoea Database cohort study. Eur Respir J 2014;44:931–41.

4. Arnardottir ES, Maislin G, Schwab RJ, et al. The interaction of obstructive sleep apnea and obesity on the inflammatory markers C-reactive protein and interleukin-6: the Icelandic Sleep Apnea Cohort. Sleep 2012;35:921–32.

5. Sateia MJ. International classification of sleep disorders. 3rd edition. Darien (IL): American Academy of Sleep Medicine; 2014.

6. Gislason T, Sunnergren O. Obstructive sleep apnea in adults. ERS Monogr 2014;65:88–105.

7. Lumeng JC, Chervin RD. Epidemiology of pediatric obstructive sleep apnea. Proc Am Thorac Soc 2008;5:242–52.

8. Guilleminault C, Querra-Salva M, Chowdhuri S, et al. Normal pregnancy, daytime sleeping, snoring and blood pressure. Sleep Med 2000;1:289–97.

9. Sarberg M, Bladh M, Josefsson A, et al. Sleepiness and sleep-disordered breathing during pregnancy. Sleep Breath 2016. [Epub ahead of print].

10. Pamidi S, Pinto LM, Marc I, et al. Maternal sleep-disordered breathing and adverse pregnancy outcomes: a systematic review and metaanalysis. Am J Obstet Gynecol 2014;210:52.e1-14.

11. Arnardottir ES, Verbraecken J, Gonçalves M, et al. Variability in recording and scoring of respiratory events during sleep in Europe: a need for uniform standards. J Sleep Res 2016;25:144–57. Available at: http://www.ncbi.nlm.nih.gov/pubmed/26365742.

12. Farré R, Montserrat JM, Rotger M, et al. Accuracy of thermistors and thermocouples as flow-measuring devices for detecting hypopnoeas. Eur Respir J 1998;11:179–82.

13. Sanders MH, Kern NB, Costantino JP, et al. Accuracy of end-tidal and transcutaneous PCO2 monitoring during sleep. Chest 1994;106:472–83.

14. Berry RB, Brooks R, Gamaldo CE, et al. The AASM manual for the scoring of sleep and associated events: rules, terminology and technical specifications, version 2.3. Darien (IL): American Academy of Sleep Medicine; 2016.

15. Vandenbussche NL, Overeem S, van Dijk JP, et al. Assessment of respiratory effort during sleep: esophageal pressure versus noninvasive monitoring techniques. Sleep Med Rev 2015;24:28–36. Available at: http://www.ncbi.nlm.nih.gov/pubmed/25644984.

16. Edmonds JC, Yang H, King TS, et al. Claustrophobic tendencies and continuous positive airway pressure therapy non-adherence in adults with obstructive sleep apnea. Heart Lung 2015;44:100–6.

17. Stuckenbrock JK, Freuschle A, Nakajima I, et al. The influence of pharyngeal and esophageal pressure measurements on the parameters of polysomnography. Eur Arch Otorhinolaryngol 2014;271:1299–304.

18. Skatvedt O, Akre H, Godtlibsen OB. Nocturnal polysomnography with and without continuous pharyngeal and esophageal pressure measurements. Sleep 1996;19:485–90.

19. Chediak AD, Demirozu MC, Nay KN. Alpha EEG sleep produced by balloon catheterization of the esophagus. Sleep 1990;13:369–70.

20. Chervin RD, Ruzicka DL, Wiebelhaus JL, et al. Tolerance of esophageal pressure monitoring during polysomnography in children. Sleep 2003;26:1022–6.

21. Kushida CA, Giacomini A, Lee MK, et al. Technical protocol for the use of esophageal manometry in the diagnosis of sleep-related breathing disorders. Sleep Med 2002;3:163–73. Available at: http://www.ncbi.nlm.nih.gov/pubmed/14592238.

22. Arnardottir ES, Isleifsson B, Agustsson JS, et al. How to measure snoring? A comparison of the microphone, cannula and piezoelectric sensor. J Sleep Res 2016;25:158–68. Available at: http://www.ncbi.nlm.nih.gov/pubmed/26553758.

23. Palombini LO, Tufik S, Rapoport DM, et al. Inspiratory flow limitation in a normal population of adults in São Paulo, Brazil. Sleep 2013;36:1663–8. Available at: http://www.ncbi.nlm.nih.gov/pubmed/24179299.

24. Guilleminault C, Stoohs R, Clerk A, et al. A cause of excessive daytime sleepiness. The upper airway resistance syndrome. Chest 1993;104:781–7.

25. Kuna ST, Benca R, Kushida CA, et al. Agreement in computer-assisted manual scoring of polysomnograms across sleep centers. Sleep 2013;36:583–9.

26. Heinzer R, Vat S, Marques-Vidal P, et al. Prevalence of sleep-disordered breathing in the general population: the HypnoLaus study. Lancet Respir Med 2015; 3:310–8.

27. Magalang UJ, Arnardottir ES, Chen NH, et al. Agreement in the scoring of respiratory events among International Sleep Centers for Home Sleep Testing. J Clin Sleep Med 2016;12:71–7.

28. Magalang UJ, Chen NH, Cistulli PA, et al, SAGIC Investigators. Agreement in the scoring of respiratory events and sleep among international sleep centers. Sleep 2013;36:591–6.

29. Guilleminault C, Lopes MC, Hagen CC, et al. The cyclic alternating pattern demonstrates increased sleep instability and correlates with fatigue and sleepiness in adults with upper airway resistance syndrome. Sleep 2007;30:641–7.

30. Svensson M, Franklin KA, Theorell-Haglöw J, et al. Daytime sleepiness relates to snoring independent of the apnea-hypopnea index in women from the general population. Chest 2008;134:919–24.

31. Tassi P, Schimchowitsch S, Rohmer O, et al. Effects of acute and chronic sleep deprivation on daytime alertness and cognitive performance of healthy snorers and non-snorers. Sleep Med 2012;13:29–35.

32. Ulfberg J, Carter N, Talbäck M, et al. Excessive daytime sleepiness at work and subjective work performance in the general population and among heavy snorers and patients with obstructive sleep apnea. Chest 1996;110:659–63.

33. Ulfberg J, Carter N, Talbäck M, et al. Headache, snoring and sleep apnoea. J Neurol 1996;243: 621–5.

34. Basoglu OK, Vardar R, Tasbakan MS, et al. Obstructive sleep apnea syndrome and gastroesophageal reflux disease: the importance of obesity and gender. Sleep Breath 2015;19:585–92.

35. Charaklias N, Mamais C, Pothula V, et al. Laryngopharyngeal reflux and primary snoring: a pilot case-control study. B-ENT 2013;9:89–93.

36. Friberg D, Gazelius B, Lindblad LE, et al. Habitual snorers and sleep apnoics have abnormal vascular reactions of the soft palatal mucosa on afferent nerve stimulation. Laryngoscope 1998;108:431–6.

37. Hagander L, Harlid R, Svanborg E. Quantitative sensory testing in the oropharynx: a means of showing nervous lesions in patients with obstructive sleep apnea and snoring. Chest 2009;136:481–9.

38. Guilleminault C, Stoohs R, Shiomi T, et al. Upper airway resistance syndrome, nocturnal blood pressure

monitoring, and borderline hypertension. Chest 1996;109:901–8.

39. Lee SA, Amis TC, Byth K, et al. Heavy snoring as a cause of carotid artery atherosclerosis. Sleep 2008; 31:1207–13.

40. Brockmann PE, Urschitz MS, Schlaud M, et al. Primary snoring in school children: prevalence and neurocognitive impairments. Sleep Breath 2012;16:23–9.

41. Jackman AR, Biggs SN, Walter LM, et al. Sleep-disordered breathing in preschool children is associated with behavioral, but not cognitive, impairments. Sleep Med 2012;13:621–31.

42. Urschitz MS, Eitner S, Guenther A, et al. Habitual snoring, intermittent hypoxia, and impaired behavior in primary school children. Pediatrics 2004;114: 1041–8.

43. Sleep-related breathing disorders in adults: recommendations for syndrome definition and measurement techniques in clinical research. The Report of an American Academy of Sleep Medicine Task Force. Sleep 1999;22:667–89.

44. Iber C, Ancoli-Israel S, Chesson AL, et al. The AASM manual for the scoring of sleep and associated events: rules, terminology, and technical specification. Version 1. Westchester (IL): American Academy of Sleep Medicine; 2007.

45. Arnardottir ES, Bjornsdottir E, Olafsdottir KA, et al. Obstructive sleep apnoea in the general population: highly prevalent but minimal symptoms. Eur Respir J 2016;47:194–202. Available at: http://www.ncbi.nlm. nih.gov/pubmed/26541533.

46. Bixler EO, Vgontzas AN, Gaines J, et al. Moderate sleep apnoea: a "silent" disorder, or not a disorder at all? Eur Respir J 2016;47:23–6.

47. Gabbay IE, Lavie P. Age- and gender-related characteristics of obstructive sleep apnea. Sleep Breath 2012;16:453–60.

48. Lavie P, Lavie L, Herer P. All-cause mortality in males with sleep apnoea syndrome: declining mortality rates with age. Eur Respir J 2005;25: 514–20.

49. Lavie P, Lavie L. Unexpected survival advantage in elderly people with moderate sleep apnoea. J Sleep Res 2009;18(4):397–403.

50. Bixler EO, Vgontzas AN, Lin HM, et al. Association of hypertension and sleep-disordered breathing. Arch Intern Med 2000;160:2289–95.

51. Sjostrom C, Lindberg E, Elmasry A, et al. Prevalence of sleep apnoea and snoring in hypertensive men: a population based study. Thorax 2002;57: 602–7.

52. Lindberg E, Taube A, Janson C, et al. A 10-year follow-up of snoring in men. Chest 1998;114: 1048–55.

53. Tam S, Woodson BT, Rotenberg B. Outcome measurements in obstructive sleep apnea: beyond the

apnea-hypopnea index. Laryngoscope 2014;124: 337–43.

54. McNicholas WT. Chronic obstructive pulmonary disease and obstructive sleep apnoea-the overlap syndrome. J Thorac Dis 2016;8:236–42.

55. Pak VM, Keenan BT, Jackson N, et al. Adhesion molecule increases in sleep apnea: beneficial effect of positive airway pressure and moderation by obesity. Int J Obes (Lond) 2014;39(3):472–9.

56. Arnardottir ES, Lim DC, Keenan BT, et al. Effects of obesity on the association between long-term sleep apnea treatment and changes in interleukin-6 levels: the Icelandic Sleep Apnea Cohort. J Sleep Res 2015;24:148–59.

57. Allan PF. High-frequency percussive ventilation: pneumotachograph validation and tidal volume analysis. Respir Care 2010;55:734–40.

58. Farré R, Montserrat JM, Navajas D. Noninvasive monitoring of respiratory mechanics during sleep. Eur Respir J 2004;24:1052–60.

59. Thurnheer R, Xie X, Bloch KE. Accuracy of nasal cannula pressure recordings for assessment of ventilation during sleep. Am J Respir Crit Care Med 2001;164:1914–9.

60. Krieger J, Kurtz D. Effects of pneumotachographic recording of breathing on sleep and respiration during sleep. Bull Eur Physiopathol Respir 1983;19: 641–4.

61. Jobin V, Rigau J, Beauregard J, et al. Evaluation of upper airway patency during Cheyne-Stokes breathing in heart failure patients. Eur Respir J 2012;40: 1523–30.

62. Montserrat JM, Farré R, Ballester E, et al. Evaluation of nasal prongs for estimating nasal flow. Am J Respir Crit Care Med 1997;155:211–5. Available at: http://www.ncbi.nlm.nih.gov/pubmed/ 9001314.

63. Ayappa I, Norman RG, Krieger AC, et al. Non-invasive detection of respiratory effort-related arousals (RERas) by a nasal cannula/pressure transducer system. Sleep 2000;23:763–71.

64. Hosselet JJ, Norman RG, Ayappa I, et al. Detection of flow limitation with a nasal cannula/pressure transducer system. Am J Respir Crit Care Med 1998;157: 1461–7.

65. Farré R, Rigau J, Montserrat JM, et al. Relevance of linearizing nasal prongs for assessing hypopneas and flow limitation during sleep. Am J Respir Crit Care Med 2001;163:494–7.

66. Montserrat JM, Farré R, Navajas D. New technologies to detect static and dynamic upper airway obstruction during sleep. Sleep Breath 2001;5: 193–206.

67. Coursey DC, Scharf SM, Johnson AT. Comparison of expiratory isovolume pressure-flow curves with the stop-flow versus the esophageal-balloon method. Respir Care 2011;56:969–75.

68. Cantineau JP, Escourrou P, Sartene R, et al. Accuracy of respiratory inductive plethysmography during wakefulness and sleep in patients with obstructive sleep apnea. Chest 1992;102: 1145–51.

69. Masa JF, Corral J, Martín MJ, et al. Assessment of thoracoabdominal bands to detect respiratory effort-related arousal. Eur Respir J 2003;22:661–7. Available at: http://www.ncbi.nlm.nih.gov/pubmed/ 14582921.

70. Sackner MA, Watson H, Belsito AS, et al. Calibration of respiratory inductive plethysmograph during natural breathing. J Appl Physiol (1985) 1989;66: 410–20.

71. Hoffstein V, Mateika S, Nash S. Comparing perceptions and measurements of snoring. Sleep 1996; 19:783–9.

72. Herzog M, Kühnel T, Bremert T, et al. The impact of the microphone position on the frequency analysis of snoring sounds. Eur Arch Otorhinolaryngol 2009; 266:1315–22.

73. Lee HK, Lee J, Kim H, et al. Snoring detection using a piezo snoring sensor based on hidden Markov models. Physiol Meas 2013;34:N41–9. Available at: http://www.ncbi.nlm.nih.gov/pubmed/ 23587724.

74. Frye RE, Doty RL. A comparison of response characteristics of airflow and pressure transducers commonly used in rhinomanometry. IEEE Trans Biomed Eng 1990;37:937–44.

75. Johns DP, Pretto JJ, Streeton JA. Measurement of gas viscosity with a Fleisch pneumotachograph. J Appl Physiol Respir Environ Exerc Physiol 1982; 53:290–3.

76. Aittokallio T, Saaresranta T, Polo-Kantola P, et al. Analysis of inspiratory flow shapes in patients with partial upper-airway obstruction during sleep. Chest 2001;119:37–44. Available at: http://www.ncbi.nlm. nih.gov/pubmed/11157582.

77. Bourjeily G, Fung JY, Sharkey KM, et al. Airflow limitations in pregnant women suspected of sleep-disordered breathing. Sleep Med 2014;15: 550–5.

78. Clark SA, Wilson CR, Satoh M, et al. Assessment of inspiratory flow limitation invasively and noninvasively during sleep. Am J Respir Crit Care Med 1998;158:713–22.

79. Agrawal S, Stone P, McGuinness K, et al. Sound frequency analysis and the site of snoring in natural and induced sleep. Clin Otolaryngol Allied Sci 2002;27:162–6.

80. Perez-Padilla JR, Slawinski E, Difrancesco LM, et al. Characteristics of the snoring noise in patients with and without occlusive sleep apnea. Am Rev Respir Dis 1993;147:635–44.

81. Lee HK, Lee J, Kim H, et al. Automatic snoring detection from nasal pressure data. Conf Proc IEEE

Eng Med Biol Soc 2013;2013:6870–2. Available at: http://www.ncbi.nlm.nih.gov/pubmed/24111323.

82. Guilleminault C, Poyares D, Palombini L, et al. Variability of respiratory effort in relation to sleep stages in normal controls and upper airway resistance syndrome patients. Sleep Med 2001;2: 397–405.

83. Masa JF, Corral J, Teran J, et al. Apnoeic and obstructive nonapnoeic sleep respiratory events. Eur Respir J 2009;34:156–61.

84. Loube DI, Andrada T, Howard RS. Accuracy of respiratory inductive plethysmography for the diagnosis of upper airway resistance syndrome. Chest 1999;115:1333–7. Available at: http://www.ncbi.nlm.nih.gov/pubmed/10334149.

85. Bloch KE, Li Y, Sackner MA, et al. Breathing pattern during sleep disruptive snoring. Eur Respir J 1997; 10:576–86.

86. Leventhall HG. Low frequency noise and annoyance. Noise Health 2004;6:59–72.

87. Beyers C. Calibration methodologies and the accuracy of acoustic data. InterNoise 2014, 43rd International Congress on Noise Control Engineering. Melbourne, Australia, November 16–19, 2014.

Definition and Importance of Autonomic Arousal in Patients with Sleep Disordered Breathing

CrossMark

Wibke Bartels, MD[a], Dana Buck, MD[a,b], Martin Glos, MSc[a],
Ingo Fietze, MD, PhD[a], Thomas Penzel, PhD[a],*

KEYWORDS

- Arousal • Autonomic arousal • Cardiovascular risk • Blood pressure • Heart rate • Hypertension
- Obstructive sleep apnea • Portapres

KEY POINTS

- Cardiovascular diseases are often found in patients with obstructive sleep apnea (OSA) because they share common risk factors such as age, gender, and metabolic disorders.
- In general, arousals indicate central nervous activation.
- In patients with sleep disordered breathing, nonphysiologic respiratory-induced arousals are predominant and cause most frequently changes in blood pressure.
- Polysomnography, including continuous blood pressure monitoring, allows insights into the cardiovascular regulation and thus allowing the qualitative and quantitative determination of autonomic arousals.

INTRODUCTION

Obstructive sleep apnea (OSA) is an increasingly common disorder that is strongly linked to cardiovascular diseases and increased mortality.[1–4] One of the most important parameters of the cardiovascular morbidity is the arterial hypertension. In a study by Peppard and colleagues,[5] OSA was a risk factor for hypertension and cardiovascular morbidity. It was reported that 40% of patients with OSA suffer from hypertension. A study on US drivers showed that 20% to 30% of patients with hypertension had OSA.[6] Hla and colleagues[7] found a significant relationship between increased blood pressure in patients with OSA and participants without OSA. The positive treatment effect of CPAP therapy on 24-hour blood pressure profiles of hypertensive patients with OSA proved the direct relation between both disorders.[8–11]

One reason that cardiovascular diseases are often found in patients with OSA is the sharing of common risk factors such as age, gender, and metabolic disorders. In addition, a causative relationship between OSA and cardiovascular diseases like hypertension and heart failure has been demonstrated.[12] Somers and associates[13,14] have argued that, among other factors, oxygen desaturation during an apnea event causes a

This study was performed within the project EU FP6 FET OPEN - 018474-2: Dynamic Analysis of Physiologic Networks (DAPHNet).
[a] Interdisciplinary Center of Sleep Medicine, Department of Cardiology, Charité Universitätsmedizin Berlin, Charité Campus Mitte, Charitéplatz 1, Berlin 10117, Germany; [b] Department of Oto-Rhino-Laryngology, Charité Universitätsmedizin Berlin, Charité Campus Mitte, Charitéplatz 1, Berlin 10117, Germany
* Corresponding author. Interdisciplinary Center of Sleep Medicine, Department of Cardiology, Charité Universitätsmedizin Berlin, Charitéplatz 1, Berlin 10117.
E-mail address: thomas.penzel@charite.de

Sleep Med Clin 11 (2016) 435–444
http://dx.doi.org/10.1016/j.jsmc.2016.08.009
1556-407X/16/© 2016 Elsevier Inc. All rights reserved.

high sympathetic activity when awake. This implies further increases in blood pressure and sympathetic activity during sleep.[13,14] Increased sympathetic activity and an elevated catecholamine level are seen day and night in patients with OSA.[15–17] Another influence exerted is the reduced baroreceptor sensitivity of patients with OSA during wakefulness and sleep.[18,19] Reduced baroreceptor sensitivity induces again an increased cardiovascular risk.[20,21] The arousal occurring after an obstructive apnea also seems to play an important role in blood pressure elevation.[22,23]

In general, arousals indicate a central nervous activation. According to the American Academy of Sleep Medicine recommendations from 2007, they are characterized by rapid electroencephalographic (EEG) frequency changes (alpha, theta) with a duration of 3 to 15 seconds,[24] but also lead to an activation of the autonomous nervous system with changes in heart rate and blood pressure. The terms used for that phenomenon are autonomic activation or autonomic arousal. During sleep, arousal could occur spontaneously as part of physiologic regulation processes, but they also could be induced by nonphysiologic stimuli like obstruction of the upper airways. Consequences of nonphysiologic arousals (>5/h) are fragmented sleep and sympathetic activation during the night as well as impairment of daytime functions. The aim of this study was to investigate the occurrence of autonomic arousal in a group of patients with sleep disordered breathing and to compare the results with a group of healthy volunteers. We wanted to establish the standardized term "autonomic arousal." With the help of visually scored arousal, we have provided a procedural definition of autonomic arousal.

MATERIALS AND METHODS
Subjects

The study protocol was approved by our ethics committee. All subjects gave informed consent. Twenty patients (10 male, 10 female; mean age, 54.4 ± 11.2 years) with OSA and 24 healthy volunteers (11 male, 13 female; mean age, 51.2 ± 8.6 years) without any kind of sleep disorders (controls) were studied in the sleep laboratory at the Charité University in Berlin. The controls were matched in age and gender to the patients. All subjects were Caucasian.

Subjects with a hypertonia in anamnesis were considered as hypertensive patients. Patients receiving antihypertensive medication had not tapered their treatment. The subjects with an Apnea/Hypopnea Index (AHI) of greater than 5 per

hour were considered to have OSA, the so-called controls had an AHI of less than 5 per hour. Subjects were excluded if they were younger than 18 years, had a body mass index (BMI) of greater than 40 kg/m[2], an alcohol or drug abuse disorder, thyroid disorder, chronic pain, neurologic or psychiatric disease, acute or severe chronic pulmonary, cardiac disease, or another severe medical disease. It was also important that the subjects did not travel across time zones or take part in another clinical study within 4 weeks before the start of our study. We excluded patients with OSA and a coexistent periodic limb movement disorder (Periodic Leg Movement Index >5 per hour).

To characterize the subjects we asked for data like body height and weight as well as medical history. Participants with a hypertension in anamnesis were considered hypertensive. A physical examination was performed.

Questionnaires

The standardized questionnaire Short Form (SF)-12, Pittsburgh Sleep Quality Index, Functional Outcomes of Sleep Questionnaire (FOSQ), and the Epworth Sleepiness Scale (ESS) were answered.

The SF-12 is the 1994 developed short version of the SF-36 (Medical Outcome Study Short Form), which detects health-related quality of life by self-assessment of physical and mental components of life quality. The Pittsburgh Sleep Quality Index is an internationally used test scrutinizing the severity of a sleep disorder. The FOSQ is a questionnaire testing the quality of life of patients with sleep disorders. The ESS is an international used method for subjective measurement of daytime sleepiness and consequent impairment.

Study Design

The subjects spent 2 subsequent nights in our sleep laboratory for recording a cardiorespiratory polysomnography (Embla Systems, Wessling, Germany) that included EEG: based on 10/20 system (C3, 01 against A2 and C4, 02 against A1), bilateral electrooculography, submental and tibialis anterior electromyography, electrocardiography, nasal airflow using nasal cannula, pulse oxyhemoglobin saturation (SpO_2) using a pulse oximeter and respiratory effort using chest and abdominal inductance belts. Especially for this study, continuous noninvasive nocturnal blood pressure measurement by Portapres system (Finapres Medical Systems BV by TNO Amsterdam, The Netherlands) was done (**Fig. 1**). Portapres is based on the arterial volume–clamp method and on the physical criteria for unloading the finger arteries.[25] For long-term monitoring of

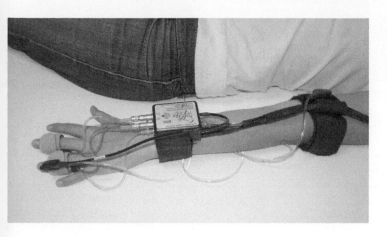

Fig. 1. Portapres system for continuous noninvasive nocturnal blood pressure measurement. (Finapres Medical Systems BV by TNO, Amsterdam, The Netherlands.)

blood pressure, there are 2 features included. The first feature allows automatic switching of the blood pressure recording between medium and ring fingers, to avoid the discomfort of long-term monitoring from a single finger. A second feature corrects the finger pressure and the hydrostatic height difference between the levels of the heart and the finger.

The blood pressure variability correlates with the intraarterial blood pressure.[26,27] The heart rate was detected from the electrocardiography in the polysomnography.

Statistical Analysis

The first night was aimed for adaptation to the sleep laboratory environment and the second night was used for visual expert analysis of sleep stages, cortical arousals, and respiration and limb movement pattern, as well as subsequent autonomic arousals to eliminate the first night effect.

Arousals were scored by using the American Academy of Sleep Medicine criteria.[24] For the characterization of autonomic arousals changes of heart rate and blood pressure were calculated within a time window of 15 seconds before versus 15 seconds after the beginning of a cortical arousal. **Figs. 2** and **3** show how we evaluated our data in a 30-second time window. We analyzed the highest and the lowest systolic and diastolic blood pressure and the highest and the lowest heart rate before and after the beginning of the arousal.

At 15 seconds before and 15 seconds after the beginning of a cortical arousal, we analyzed the

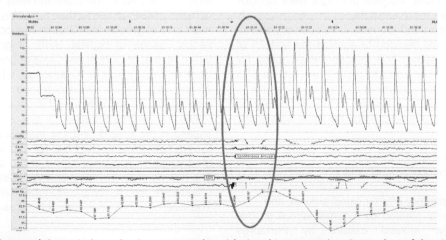

Fig. 2. A 30-second time window of polysomnography with signal interpretation. Screenshot of the visual arousal scoring: 15 seconds before versus 15 seconds after the beginning of an (electroencephalography) arousal (*center, mark*). Top, The signals of the blood pressure. Bottom, The heart rate (detected from the electrocardiograph). The mark on the left side shows a calibration of the Portapres system. REM, rapid eye movement.

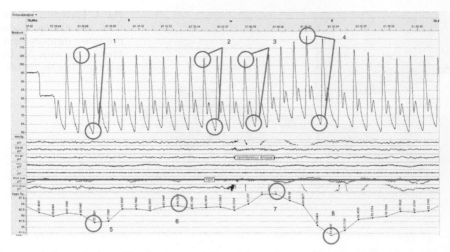

Fig. 3. A 30-second time window of polysomnography with scoring results. The circles above show the blood pressure related to the arousal: 1, highest systolic and diastolic blood pressure before the arousal; 2, lowest systolic and diastolic blood pressure before the arousal; 3, lowest systolic and diastolic blood pressure after the arousal; 4, highest systolic and diastolic blood pressure after the arousal. The circles below show the heart rate related to the arousals; 5, lowest heart rate before the arousal; 6, highest heart rate before the arousal; 7, highest heart rate after the arousal; 8, lowest heart rate after the arousal.

normal blood pressure and heart rate, which are restored within 15 seconds from the initial perturbation (eg, cortical arousal).[28,29] In addition, it is unusual that many second arousals are seen during that short period of time. In case that a second arousal was seen during the 15 seconds after 1 arousal we did not analyze those arousal because it is difficult to evaluate if the physiologic reaction belongs to the first or the second arousal.

Because of the missing of guidelines for the classification of arousal severities, we decided to divide arousals in different categories corresponding to the classification of OSA severities. Subjects with 50 or more arousals per night were considered to have more arousals.

If more than 150 arousals were seen in patients with OSA, we decided to analyze the first 25 of each sleep stage. This selection was chosen for practical reasons and to prevent the results of a particular patient dominating the overall results.

Arousals were classified further according to their causes as evaluated by the other biosignals:

1. Respiratory arousal;
2. Limb movement arousal;
3. Spontaneous arousal; and
4. Others:
   a. Respiratory effort–related arousal; and
   b. Arousal caused by external stimuli (in this study: arousal caused by Portapres impact = Portapres arousal).

The mean arterial blood pressure (MBP = diastolic pressure + 1/3 [systolic pressure – diastolic pressure]) was calculated. To compare the cardiovascular response to the different arousal categories of the patients with OSA and the controls, we defined a change in the MBP in the following way: increase, greater than 5 mm Hg; decrease, less than -5 mm Hg; and unchanged, ±5 mm Hg. The change in heart rate was also defined as follows: increase, greater than 3 bpm; decrease less than, -3 bpm; and unchanged, ±3 bpm. The definition of heart rate change is based on the study by Basner and colleagues,[30] who also examined changes in heart rate after arousal.

For our analysis we defined an autonomic arousal as follows. An autonomic arousal in sleep is a change of highest MBP of greater than 5 mm Hg, of highest heart rate of greater than 3 bpm or a contemporaneous change of highest MBP of greater than 5 mm Hg and of highest heart rate of greater than 3 bpm within a period of 30 seconds, which means 15 seconds before an occurrence (eg, cortical arousal) and 15 seconds after this occurrence.

For the characterization of the subjects, we assessed the means and the standard deviation (SD) in both groups. The t test for normally distributed variables was used to find group differences. The non parametric χ^2 test and the Mann–Whitney U test were used to compare independent samples. The level of significance was defined as $P \leq .05$.

RESULTS

Age and gender were matched (**Table 1**). The BMI was significantly higher in patients ($P = .039$). Nine

Table 1
Subjects characteristics

	Patients with OSA	Controls
No. of subjects	20	24
Gender		
Female	10	13
Male	10	11
Age (y)		
Range	41–76	28–69
Mean ± SD	54.4 ± 11.2	51.2 ± 8.6
Body mass index (kg/m^2), mean ± SD	29.35 ± 5.08	24.4 ± 2.9
Hypertension, n (%)	8 (40)	1 (4.2)
Antihypertensive medication, n (%)	7 (35)	1 (4.2)
Questionnaires (no. of patients), mean ± SD		
PSQI	7.9 ± 4	3.3 ± 1.36
FOSQ	16.8 ± 3.2	19.5 ± 0.6
SF 12 (physical)	46.2 ± 9.1	54.1 ± 2.4
SF 12 (mental)	48.5 ± 12.8	56.2 ± 2.2
ESS	6.83 ± 4.1	4.8 ± 2.5
AHI (/h), mean ± SD	22.48 ± 21.82	0.8 ± 1.13
Arousal, mean ± SD	92.25 ± 63.02	23.35 ± 46.5
Arousal (all)	2151	1089
Respiratory arousal, n (%)	1557 (72.4)	33 (3)
LM arousal, n (%)	268 (12.5)	319 (29.3)
Spontaneous arousal, n (%)	228 (10.6)	663 (60.9)
RERA, n (%)	84 (3.9)	37 (3.4)
Portapres-induced arousal, n (%)	14 (0.7)	37 (3.4)

Abbreviations: AHI, Apnea/Hypopnea Index; FOSQ, Functional Outcomes of Sleep Questionnaire; LM, limb movement; OSA, obstructive sleep apnea; PSQI, Pittsburgh Sleep Quality Index; RERA, respiratory effort–related arousal; SD, standard deviation; SF-12, Short Form-12.

patients with OSA and just 1 control were obese (BMI >30 kg/m^2). There were significantly more patients with a hypertension in the OSA patients group (8 patients with OSA) than in the healthy volunteer group (1 healthy volunteer; $P = .002$; **Table 2**). There were also significantly more hypertensives in patients with more arousal (>50 arousals per night) than in patients with less arousal (<50 arousals per night; $P = .009$; **Table 3**). Significant differences were found between both groups in the questionnaires Pittsburgh Sleep Quality Index ($P<.001$), FOSQ ($P<.001$), and in the physical component of SF 12 ($P = .004$). No

Table 2
Comparison hypertension and OSA categories

Severity Degree	AHI [/h]	Hypertension, n (%) Yes	No
No OSA	<5	1 (11.1)	23 (65.7)
Nonsevere OSA	5 to <15	3 (33.3)	6 (17.1)
Moderate OSA	15 to <30	2 (22.2)	4 (11.4)
Severe OSA	>30	3 (33.3)	2 (5.7)

Abbreviations: AHI, Apnea/Hypopnea Index; OSA, obstructive sleep apnea.

Table 3
Comparison hypertension and arousal frequency

Arousal Frequency	Hypertension, n (%) Yes	No
≤50	0 (0)	18 (51.4)
51–100	4 (44.4)	13 (37.1)
101–149	3 (33.3)	2 (5.7)
≥150	2 (22.2)	2 (5.7)

differences were seen between both groups in ESS (P = NS) and in the mental component of SF-12 (P = NS). Most patients with OSA had no daytime sleepiness, some of them had a nonsevere OSA (AHI 5–15), some a moderate OSA (AHI 15–30), and some a severe OSA (AHI >30). In only 3 patients with moderate and severe OSA was an indication of increased daytime sleepiness found. One patient with a nonsevere OSA had indications of a pathologic daytime sleepiness.

A higher AHI and more arousals were seen in patients with OSA. In OSA group 2151 EEG arousals (type: 72% respiratory, 13% limb movement, 11% spontaneous, 4% other) and in group of controls 1089 EEG arousals (type: 3% respiratory, 29% limb movement, 61% spontaneous, 7% other) were scored. For the sake of completeness, 8 second arousals were detected during the short time window of 15 seconds after one EEG arousal, but they were not included in analysis.

The highest systolic blood pressure, diastolic blood pressure, MBP, and heart rate increased significantly after an arousal in both groups ($P<.001$; Table 4). The lowest systolic blood pressure, diastolic blood pressure, MBP, and heart rate increased mostly not significantly after an arousal in both groups. In patients with OSA the highest MBP increased from 93.1 ± 13.5 to 101.5 ± 12.7 mm Hg and the highest heart rate changed from 70.3 ± 7.8 to 75.9 ± 7.6 bpm. In the control group, the highest MBP increased from 87.0 ± 12.4 to 94.8 ± 13.0 mm Hg and the highest heart rate increased from 67.3 ± 8.9 to 73.2 ± 8.4 bpm. Comparing patients with healthy volunteers, there are differences between the absolute blood pressure and heart rate level, but these findings are not significant (P = NS).

Arousals were found most frequent with increases in highest MBP (65% of cases) and by increases in highest heart rate (62%) in both subject groups (Fig. 4A, B). When combining the highest MBP and the highest heart rate an increase was seen in 76% of the cases (Fig. 4C). Furthermore, there was a positive correlation between arousal-induced highest MBP and highest heart rate changes (r = 0.27; $P<.001$; Fig. 5).

Respiratory arousals are seen predominantly in the patient group and spontaneous arousals are seen predominantly in the control group (Fig. 6). Respiratory arousals are predominantly associated with an increase of highest MBP in both groups. Of all arousal categories, respiratory arousal caused in 73.5% of cases an increase of highest MBP in the patient group. In the control group, Portapres arousal caused most often (75%) an increase in highest MBP, followed by respiratory arousal, causing an increase in 73.1% of cases. Spontaneous arousal caused an increase

Table 4
Blood pressure and heart rate change after an arousal

	Patients with OSA			Controls		
	Before Arousal, Mean ± SD	After Arousal, Mean ± SD	P	Before Arousal Mean ± SD	After Arousal Mean ± SD	P
Lowest SBP (mm Hg)	118.7 ± 16.9	121.4 ± 17.4	.013	110.8 ± 14.7	111.9 ± 15.1	.212
Lowest DBP (mm Hg)	67.7 ± 12.4	68.2 ± 12.6	.372	62.2 ± 10.3	61.6 ± 10.5	.162
Lowest MBP (mm Hg)	84.7 ± 13.0	85.9 ± 13.0	.075	78.4 ± 11.1	78.4 ± 11.1	.909
Highest SBP (mm Hg)	135.6 ± 18.4	150.3 ± 18.1	<.001	126.8 ± 16.7	141.5 ± 19.1	<.001
Highest DBP (mm Hg)	71.8 ± 12.9	77.1 ± 12.9	<.001	67.2 ± 11.4	71.4 ± 11.7	<.001
Highest MBP (mm Hg)	93.1 ± 13.5	101.5 ± 12.7	<.001	87.0 ± 12.4	94.8 ± 13.0	<.001
Lowest HR (bpm)	59.3 ± 7.9	59.2 ± 7.8	.903	58.0 ± 8.3	57.2 ± 8.2	.043
Highest HR (bpm)	70.3 ± 7.8	75.9 ± 7.6	<.001	67.3 ± 8.9	73.2 ± 8.4	<.001

Abbreviations: AHI, Apnea/Hypopnea Index; DBP, diastolic blood pressure; HR, heart rate; MBP, mean arterial blood pressure; OSA, obstructive sleep apnea; SBP, systolic blood pressure.

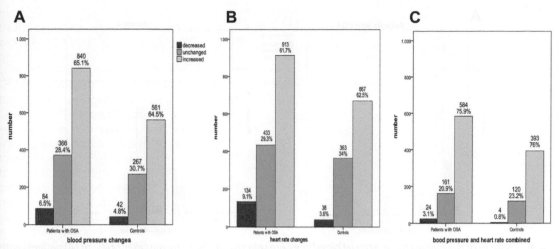

Fig. 4. Changes of the highest mean arterial blood pressure and the highest heart rate after the arousal. (*A*) Blood pressure changes. (*B*) Heart rate changes. (*C*) Blood pressure and heart rate changes combined. OSA, obstructive sleep apnea.

in 60.5% of the cases in patients with OSA and in 66.9% of the cases in the controls.

DISCUSSION

In patients with sleep disordered breathing, the nonphysiologic respiratory-induced arousals are predominant and cause most frequently changes in blood pressure. The accumulated activation of the cardiovascular system during sleep has negative consequences. We found significant differences in hypertension in participants with more and with less arousal.

SUBJECTS CHARACTERISTICS

The 20 patients with OSA and the 24 controls were compared; age and gender were roughly the same because of careful matching during recruitment. The BMI of the patients with OSA was significantly higher compared with the controls. Obesity is often seen in patients with OSA. In obese individuals, anatomic and functional considerations of the pharyngeal airway, central obesity, and leptin interact in the development of OSA.[31] In fact, weight loss or a change in lifestyle and nutrition is an important therapy for OSA; weight loss causes an improvement of OSA severity.[32,33] The

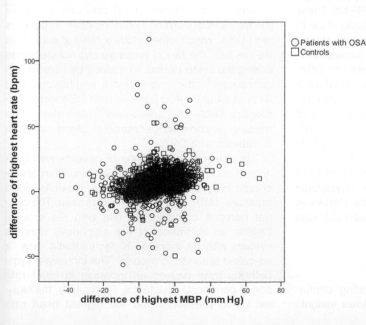

Fig. 5. The relation between the difference of highest mean arterial blood pressure (MBP) and highest heart rate. OSA, obstructive sleep apnea.

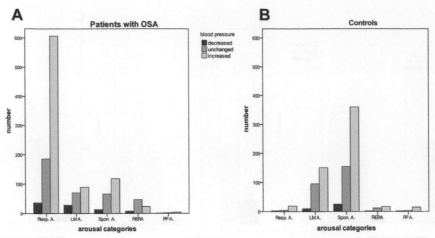

Fig. 6. Changes of the highest mean arterial blood pressure split to different arousal categories for (A) patients with obstructive sleep apnea (OSA) and (B) controls. LM A., limb movement arousal; PPA., arousal caused by external stimuli; Resp. A., respiratory arousal; RERA, respiratory effort–related arousal; Spon. A., spontaneous arousal.

obesity also plays an important role in the development of cardiovascular diseases in patients with OSA.[34] There were significantly more hypertensives in the group of patients than in the group of controls. There were also significantly more hypertensives in participants with more arousal than in participants with less arousal. OSA is strongly linked to cardiovascular diseases such as hypertension as well as increased mortality.[1–4]

In contrast with other findings, for example, from Johns,[35] we found no correlation between the severity of OSA and an elevated daytime sleepiness on the ESS. Our findings conform with a study from Bausmer and colleagues,[36] where also no correlation was found between the ESS and the AHI of 130 patients with OSA and upper airway pathology. The quality of life was limited (FOSQ, SF-12). These findings reflect the constriction in the quality of life, to which a "good sleep" belongs. The daytime sleepiness seems to be not as important as expected.

A higher AHI and more arousal caused by OSA, especially respiratory arousals, were seen in the patient group. It is important that patients with OSA and a coexistent periodic leg movement- index of greater than 5 per hour were excluded therefore not so many leg movement arousals were seen in patients with OSA. Otherwise, the frequent occurrence of respiratory arousal in patients with OSA was shown. In the group of controls, physiologic spontaneous arousals dominated. The Portapres can induce arousal by external stimulation, although these events are rare.

AUTONOMIC AROUSAL

The use of polysomnography, including continuous blood pressure monitoring, allows insights into the cardiovascular regulation and thus allows qualitative and quantitative determination of autonomic arousals. Autonomic arousals are presented by increases in blood pressure and heart rate. We studied autonomic arousal so that we could recommend a definition. Therefore, we compared changes in blood pressure and heart rate before and after arousals in patients with OSA and in controls.

The blood pressure and the heart rate of the patients with OSA were higher than those of the controls, but these findings were not significant. As mentioned, hypertension in the group of patients with OSA may explain the higher blood pressure during the night; hypertensives have a higher blood pressure profile by definition. Another reason for the higher blood pressure could be the frequent occurrence of 'nondipper' in patients with OSA, which other studies have shown. This means that the blood pressure did not decrease during the sleep period. In a study by Loredo and colleagues,[37] the investigators emphasized that 84% of 44 untreated patients with OSA were nondippers. Grote and colleagues[38] refer also to the missing physiologic decrease in blood pressure in patients with OSA.

The physiologic reactions of patients with OSA and of controls after arousal were similar: an increase in systolic blood pressure, diastolic blood pressure, MBP, and heart rate was seen. The central nervous activation in line with the arousal causes an activation of the autonomic nervous system with an increase in sympathetic tone, a so-called autonomic arousal. The increased sympathetic tone causes an increase in heart rate and in peripheral resistance. Particularly, the highest blood pressures and the highest heart rate increased significantly in both groups. It is important that there were no differences in the regulation of the systolic blood pressure, diastolic blood pressure, and MBP. The differences were more seen in the lowest and the highest blood pressures and the lowest and the highest heart rate. Arousals were presented mostly by increases in highest MBP and by increases in highest heart rate in both groups. When combining the highest MBP and the highest heart rate, an increase was seen in 76% of cases.

With our results, we showed that our initial suggestion for the definition of autonomic arousal is useful. It is important to develop automatic data interpretation for the variations of parameters and for the definition. Perhaps it would be possible to predict cortical arousals out of autonomic arousals or to draw conclusions of cardiovascular morbidity from the autonomic arousals. To simplify the polysomnography would be time and cost effective.

These findings contribute to a better understanding of the relationship between sleep disordered breathing, autonomic arousal, and cardiovascular consequences.

REFERENCES

1. Golbin JM, Somers VK, Caples SM. Obstructive sleep apnea, cardiovascular disease, and pulmonary hypertension. Proc Am Thorac Soc 2008;5: 200–6.

2. Lavie P, Lavie L. Cardiovascular morbidity and mortality in obstructive sleep apnea. Curr Pharm Des 2008;14:3466–73.

3. Parish JM, Somers VK. Obstructive sleep apnea and cardiovascular disease. Mayo Clin Proc 2004;79: 1036–46.

4. Punjabi NM, Caffo BS, Goodwin JL, et al. Sleep-disordered breathing and mortality: a prospective cohort study. PLoS Med 2009;6:e1000132.

5. Peppard PE, Young T, Palta M, et al. Prospective study of the association between sleep-disordered breathing and hypertension. N Engl J Med 2000; 342:1378–84.

6. Stoohs RA, Bingham LA, Itoi A, et al. Sleep and sleep-disordered breathing in commercial long-haul truck drivers. Chest 1995;107:1275–82.

7. Hla KM, Young TB, Bidwell T, et al. Sleep apnea and hypertension. A population-based study. Ann Intern Med 1994;120:382–8.

8. Becker HF, Jerrentrup A, Ploch T, et al. Effect of nasal continuous positive airway pressure treatment on blood pressure in patients with obstructive sleep apnea. Circulation 2003;1:68–73.

9. Faccenda JF, Mackay TW, Boon NA, et al. Randomized placebo-controlled trial of continuous positive airway pressure on blood pressure in the sleep apnea-hypopnea syndrome. Am J Respir Crit Care Med 2001;163:344–8.

10. Hui DS, To KW, Ko FW, et al. Nasal CPAP reduces systemic blood pressure in patients with obstructive sleep apnoea and mild sleepiness. Thorax 2006;61: 1083–90.

11. Pepperell JC, Ramdassingh-Dow S, Crosthwaite N, et al. Ambulatory blood pressure after therapeutic and subtherapeutic nasal continuous positive airway pressure for obstructive sleep apnoea: a randomised parallel trial. Lancet 2002;359:204–10.

12. Devulapally K, Pongonis R Jr, Khayat R. OSA: the new cardiovascular disease: part II: overview of cardiovascular diseases associated with obstructive sleep apnea. Heart Fail Rev 2009;14:155–64.

13. Somers VK, Mark AL, Zavala DC, et al. Contrasting effects of hypoxia and hypercapnia on ventilation and sympathetic activity in humans. J Appl Physiol (1985) 1989;67:2101–6.

14. Somers VK, Dyken ME, Clary MP, et al. Sympathetic neural mechanisms in obstructive sleep apnea. J Clin Invest 1995;96:1897–904.

15. Elmasry A, Lindberg E, Hedner J, et al. Obstructive sleep apnoea and urine catecholamines in hypertensive males: a population-based study. Eur Respir J 2002;19:511–7.

16. Leuenberger U, Jacob E, Sweer L, et al. Surges of muscle sympathetic nerve activity during obstructive apnea are linked to hypoxemia. J Appl Physiol (1985) 1995;79:581–8.

17. Ziegler MG, Nelesen R, Mills P, et al. Sleep apnea, norepinephrine-release rate, and daytime hypertension. Sleep 1997;20:224–31.

18. Cooper VL, Bowker CM, Pearson SB, et al. Effects of simulated obstructive sleep apnoea on the human carotid baroreceptor-vascular resistance reflex. J Physiol 2004;557(Pt 3):1055–65.

19. Parati G, Di Renzo M, Bonsignore MR, et al. Autonomic cardiac regulation in obstructive sleep apnea syndrome: evidence from spontaneous baroreflex analysis during sleep. J Hypertens 1997;15(12 Pt 2):1621–6.

20. Cooper VL, Pearson SB, Bowker CM, et al. Interaction of chemoreceptor and baroreceptor reflexes by hypoxia and hypercapnia - a mechanism for promoting hypertension in obstructive sleep apnoea. J Physiol 2005;568(Pt 2):677–87.

21. La Rovere MT, Bigger JT Jr, Marcus FI, et al. Baroreflex sensitivity and heart-rate variability in prediction of total cardiac mortality after myocardial infarction. ATRAMI (autonomic tone and reflexes after myocardial infarction) Investigators. Lancet 1998;351:478–84.

22. Davies RJ, Belt PJ, Roberts SJ, et al. Arterial blood pressure responses to graded transient arousal from sleep in normal humans. J Appl Physiol (1985) 1993;74:1123–30.

23. Yoon IY, Jeong DU. Degree of arousal is most correlated with blood pressure reactivity during sleep in obstructive sleep apnea. J Korean Med Sci 2001; 16:707–11.

24. Iber C, Ancoli-Israel S, Chesson A, et al. The AASM manual for the scoring of sleep and associated events: rules, terminology and technical specifications. 1st edition. Westchester (IL): American Academy of Sleep Medicine; 2007.

25. Wesseling KH, de Wit B, van der Hoeven GMA, et al. Physiocal, calibrating finger vascular physiology for Finapres. Homeostasis 1995;36:67–82.

26. Parati G, Casadei R, Groppelli A, et al. Comparison of finger and intra-arterial blood pressure monitoring at rest and during laboratory testing. Hypertension 1989;13(6 Pt 1):647–55.

27. Parati G, Ongaro G, Bilo G, et al. Non-invasive beat-to-beat blood pressure monitoring: new developments. Blood Press Monit 2003;8:31–6.

28. Silvani A, Magosso E, Bastianini S, et al. Mathematical modeling of cardiovascular coupling: central autonomic commands and baroreflex control. Auton Neurosci 2011;162(1–2):66–71.

29. Sforza E, Jouny C, Ibanez V. Cardiac activation during arousal in humans: further evidence for hierarchy in the arousal response. Clin Neurophysiol 2000; 111(9):1611–9.

30. Basner M, Griefahn B, Muller U, et al. An ECG-based algorithm for the automatic identification of autonomic activations associated with cortical arousal. Sleep 2007;10:1349–61.

31. Gami AS, Caples SM, Somers VK. Obesity and obstructive sleep apnea. Endocrinol Metab Clin North Am 2003;32:869–94.

32. Newman AB, Foster G, Givelber R, et al. Progression and regression of sleep-disordered breathing with changes in weight: the Sleep Heart Health Study. Arch Intern Med 2005;165:2408–13.

33. Romero-Corral A, Caples SM, Lopez-Jimenez F, et al. Interactions between obesity and obstructive sleep apnea: implications for treatment. Chest 2010;137:711–9.

34. Ramar K, Caples SM. Cardiovascular consequences of obese and nonobese obstructive sleep apnea. Med Clin North Am 2010;94:465–78.

35. Johns MW. A new method for measuring daytime sleepiness: the Epworth sleepiness Scale. Sleep 1991;14:540–5.

36. Bausmer U, Gouveris H, Selivanova O, et al. Correlation of the Epworth Sleepiness Scale with respiratory sleep parameters in patients with sleep-related breathing disorders and upper airway pathology. Eur Arch Otorhinolaryngol 2010;267:1645–8.

37. Loredo JS, Ancoli-Israel S, Dimsdale JE. Sleep quality and blood pressure dipping in obstructive sleep apnea. Am J Hypertens 2001;14(9 Pt 1): 887–92.

38. Grote L, Heitmann J, Köhler U, et al. Assessment of the nocturnal blood pressure relative to sleep stages in patients with obstructive sleep apnea. Z Kardiol 1996;85(Suppl 3):112–4.

Telemedicine Applications in Sleep Disordered Breathing
Thinking Out of the Box

Johan Verbraecken, MD, PhD

KEYWORDS

- Telemedicine • Sleep disordered breathing • Technology • Monitoring

KEY POINTS

- Telemedicine encompasses the use of information and communication technology (telephone, video, Internet, satellite, cloud) to deliver health care at a distance.
- Diagnostic telemedicine applications include telemonitored polysomnography, long-term polygraphic monitoring, and remote continuous positive airway pressure (CPAP) titration.
- Telemedicine allows clinicians to remotely monitor CPAP adherence and compliance and fine-tune CPAP settings.
- Patient counseling, as well as therapy reinforcement by combining and integrating psychoeducational interventions and telemonitoring, is feasible.
- Barriers like patient's and physician's cooperation, privacy concerns, financial barriers, technological barriers, and quality concerns have to be overcome.

INTRODUCTION

The popularity of technology is increasing in nearly every field, and sleep medicine is no exception. Telemedicine as a means of remote patient-physician interaction is growing and virtual consultations with sleep specialists are feasible.[1] The potential benefits of telemedicine include improved access to health care, reduced waiting time for appointments, and increased adherence to chronic illness treatment plans.[2] Because many sleep disorders, particularly sleep apnea, are chronic conditions, and require a continuous treatment and monitoring of therapy success, telematic communications and new information technologies could be useful to establish diagnostic and therapeutic strategies. It is important to install cost-efficient technologies for an initial simple diagnosis, rapid treatment initiation, and

for long-term monitoring of treatment adherence and compliance, providing the possibility for patients to avoid traveling.[3] A substantial proportion of patients are willing to consider telemedicine as an option for their care. In such settings, in case of insufficient adherence or compliance, device dysfunction, or subjective problems, alerts can be generated and sent to the health professional, who can react rapidly and focus on the patient's needs.

In this article, telemedicine solutions in sleep disordered breathing are reviewed, with emphasis on adherence and compliance monitoring:

- Diagnostic telemedicine applications: telemonitored polysomnography, long-term polygraphic monitoring.
- Remote continuous positive airway pressure (CPAP) titration.

Department of Pulmonary Medicine, Multidisciplinary Sleep Disorders Centre, Antwerp University Hospital, University of Antwerp, Wilrijkstraat 10, Edegem, Antwerp 2650, Belgium
E-mail address: johan.verbraecken@uza.be

Sleep Med Clin 11 (2016) 445–459
http://dx.doi.org/10.1016/j.jsmc.2016.08.007
1556-407X/16/© 2016 The Author. Published by Elsevier Inc. This is an open access article under the CC BY-NC-ND
license (http://creativecommons.org/licenses/by-nc-nd/4.0/)

- Monitoring of CPAP adherence and compliance:
  - Standard care
  - Remote monitoring and fine-tuning therapy
- Patient counseling and therapy reinforcement by combining and integrating the most promising elements of both psychoeducational interventions and technological innovations.
- Barriers in the implementation of telemedicine are also highlighted.

DIAGNOSTIC TELEMEDICINE APPLICATIONS
Telemonitored Polysomnography

Telemonitored polysomnography (PSG) is designed to overcome the disadvantages of home recordings and could provide an organizational solution to the overloading of specialized sleep centers. Dedicated technicians regularly verify, at a distance, the quality of the PSG recordings by means of periodic access to the PSG monitoring device. From a telemonitoring control panel, they are able to insert comments in the recording; adjust transducer gain; and, in the event of an artifact or an undesirable accident, inform the patient by telephone.[4] However, evidence on the efficacy of telemonitored PSG is weak. Gagnadoux and colleagues[5] reported that PSG performed in a local hospital and telemonitored by a sleep laboratory was clearly superior to unattended home PSG. Kristo and colleagues[6] proposed a telemedicine protocol for the online transfer of PSG data from a remote site to a centralized sleep laboratory, which provided a cost-saving approach for the diagnosis of obstructive sleep apnea (OSA). Their system was based on the transmission of data using an Internet file transfer protocol (FTP), which is the conventional system for file transfer. Kayyali and colleagues[7] presented a new compact telemetry-based sleep monitor, consisting of a 14-channel wearable wireless monitor and a cell phone–based gateway to transfer data, including video, in real time from the patient's home to a remote sleep center. The monitor can easily be worn and transported, and it offers reliable recordings. The receiver is a separate unit connected with the back of the display. Internal Bluetooth receivers, usually included in laptops, can also be used instead of a dedicated external Bluetooth receiver. A major problem encountered with home sleep studies is the potential loss of data in about 4.7% to 20% of the cases, which results in lower than expected cost savings.[8] Using Sleepbox technology (Medatec, Brussels, Belgium), a wireless system able to communicate with the polysomnograph and with Internet through a WiFi/3G interface, and

communicating via Skype, the investigators were able to deliver recordings with excellent quality in 90% of the cases.[9] This finding suggests an interesting way to decrease the failure rate of home sleep studies, although it is still problematic, and some technical aspects need to be improved. Pelletier-Fleury and colleagues[10] comparatively evaluated the cost and effectiveness of PSG telemonitoring and PSG by conventional unsupervised home monitoring, and showed that remote telemonitoring made the procedure clearly superior from a technical point of view and was preferred by the patients. The cost of PSG telemonitoring was US$244, whereas the cost of PSG with conventional unsupervised home monitoring was US$153. The health care infrastructure savings have to be taken into account as well. For example, by adding up the working days that the patients did not lose and the round-trip travel costs they avoided, it can be estimated that the real cost would be similar or lower than that of conventional PSG.[3] Masa and colleagues[11] compared the costs made between device transportation and telematic transmission of data, with comparable results. Having devices moved by a transportation company or sent telematically as raw data proved cost-effective and equally beneficial. This finding opens the possibility of application among patients who live a long way from the hospital or those with limited mobility. Fields and colleagues[12] showed the feasibility of a comprehensive, telemedicine-based OSA evaluation and management pathway compared with a more traditional, in-person care model. They combined video consultation for intake with home sleep testing using a type 3 portable monitor with remote download, and automatic CPAP (autoCPAP) titration with wireless modem technology. Patient satisfaction, CPAP adherence and compliance, and improvement in quality of life were similar in both groups.

Long-Term Polygraphic Monitoring

In clinical practice, the use of PSG is a standard procedure to assess sleep disordered breathing. However, PSG is not suitable for chronic monitoring in the home environment. New telemedicine applications have become available using a home appliance as a precautionary measure for monitoring snoring and OSA. Seo and colleagues[13] developed a nonintrusive health-monitoring home system to monitor patients' electrocardiogram (ECG) results, weight, motor activity, and snoring. Choi and colleagues[14] proposed a ubiquitous health-monitoring system in a bedroom, which monitors the ECG, body movements, and snoring with nonconscious sensors. Böhning and colleagues[15] evaluated the feasibility of night-time pulse-oximetry telemedicine to screen patients at risk for OSA. They concluded that the technique seemed to be suitable and cost-effective, with high sensitivity and specificity. This approach can be applied in a telemedicine referral network for early diagnosis of OSA, and the reading could be transmitted to the relevant sleep laboratory, examined, and the results returned to the referring physician.[16]

THERAPEUTIC TELEMEDICINE APPLICATIONS
Remote Continuous Positive Airway Pressure Titration

An exploratory study was set up to perform real-time titration of domiciliary CPAP.[17] The novelty of this approach is that a telemetry unit is connected to a commercially available CPAP device to allow a low-cost, 2-way communication channel in real time between the sleep laboratory technician and the CPAP device in the patient's home. The approach requires no special telemedicine approach, nor does it require the patient's active cooperation or any kind of communication infrastructure (computer or the Internet) in the patient's home.

Monitoring of Continuous Positive Airway Pressure Compliance and Adherence

Continuous positive airway pressure adherence and compliance

Because CPAP is a self-administered treatment, its efficacy is critically dependent on the patient's willingness to use the device and apply the nasal mask during sleep, regardless of how well a CPAP machine corrects apnea. In this context, the term adherence is used to describe continued use of the machine (ie, uptake), whereas compliance expresses the use of CPAP for a certain amount of time.[18] However, these terms are often inadequately used and interchangeable. A user is defined as a patient who uses the device for greater than 4 hours per night. Commonly used definitions of adequate compliance are usage of greater than 4 hours per night for 70% of days or greater than 4 hours per night for more than 5 d/wk.[19,20] Different studies have shown that the rates of CPAP use are between 30% and 60%. Note that patients who become nonadherent in the first days of CPAP treatment generally remain nonadherent.[21] Without optimal CPAP use, patients fail to achieve the full cardiovascular and symptomatic benefits of therapy.

Hence, compliance for CPAP should be regarded as the main determinant for success.[18]

Self-reports are an inaccurate tool to determine compliance with CPAP therapy for OSA. Trying to estimate daily use time by simply questioning how many hours a night the patient uses the device generally results in a considerable misestimation of mean treatment time per night, because the patient is likely to provide the number of hours of CPAP use solely for the nights it was worn. Including the question about the number of nights on CPAP per week makes self-reports of CPAP use more accurate. This discrepancy may be attributed to not using the machine when traveling, during episodes of upper airway infection, or during self-prescribed treatment vacations from time to time. Another explanation is that many patients do not reestablish CPAP after the first awakening in the morning. Altogether, a more objective approach is mandatory. At present, CPAP usage is assessed by using time meters or more sophisticated devices that measure both run time and pressure delivery. It is increasingly accepted in sleep medicine that good compliance consists of 4 hours or more of CPAP per night and 70% of the nights, and that this is needed to achieve optimal symptom control.[22,23] The literature shows that between 29% and 83% of patients do not meet the criteria for good compliance because of removing CPAP early in the night and/or discontinuing use. Patients' perceptions of CPAP within the first weeks of using the machine affect the long-term results of CPAP adherence and compliance.[24] Objective compliance can be obtained from the average number of hours of running of the machine per 24 hours, calculated from the built-in time counter of the device, but, preferably, effective compliance is assessed based on the time spent at the prescribed effective pressure per night, using a pressure monitor coupled with a microprocessor.[25] Microprocessors use an algorithm for the detection of mask-on pressure. The variable component of the pressure signal given by the pressure transducer is analyzed in order to determine whether the patient is breathing into the mask. Reductions in therapeutic pressure greater than 2 to 5 cm and lasting longer than 10 seconds can be documented as mask-off events. Thus, the duration of therapeutic pressure delivery per day (also referred to as mask time) and number of missed days of use can be determined. From these data, several parameters can be calculated (percentage of days when CPAP was used; percentage of days when CPAP was used for >4 hours; mean daily use; mean daily use on days CPAP was used), including mean delivery pressure and residual apnea-hypopnea index (AHI). This approach is usually described as CPAP adherence tracking, although the term

CPAP compliance tracking might be more applicable.[26] Modern CPAP devices can be interfaced with a computer in the physician's office or home setting to download data. Newer modems can interface with the CPAP unit and the integrated chip to facilitate the reporting of remote data and reduce the need for face-to-face visits.[27] These modems may be used as augmentation to therapy for adherent patients or to identify and assist non-adherent patients. In addition, smart cards can be inserted into slots in the CPAP devices to imprint the data. These cards are then transported to the appropriate professional in a variety of ways, including the use of mail carriers or other modes, to reduce the need for direct patient travel for routine compliance and adherence reporting. These cards track usage hours, mask leak (liters per second), pressure, snoring, and AHI, and may assist sleep technicians, specialists, and home care providers with feedback on efficacy data to determine effective therapy and to measure outcomes. AHI measurements by some machines have been shown to be highly correlated with the measures recorded by PSG.[28] However, there are known problems with loss of data and failure of recording systems (primarily smart cards).[26,29] An evolutionary development in the collection and reporting of adherence and compliance data is wireless and Internet technologies to transmit clinical data to remote sites.[27] The powerful ability to track daily CPAP use facilitates rapid detection of decreased compliance, nonadherence, or suboptimal apnea correction to reduce the burden and risks and ensure cost-efficacy.

Standard follow-up

The patient should be seen by a qualified sleep professional to assess CPAP usage (hours of use and hours of application), to check the machine settings, and to ensure the interface (mask, pillows, and so forth) is in good condition. Short-term and long-term follow-up are crucial to adherence and compliance, but monitoring efficacy is also critical to adherence, compliance, and successful therapy. The results of the hours/usage monitor should be discussed and the need to be adherent to the prescribed treatment reinforced. An annual office visit should also be scheduled to check all the equipment and the hours/usage and to replace masks. Changes in the patient's overall condition may warrant a change in CPAP pressure (ie, weight gain may allow a higher CPAP setting or vice versa). In one study, compliance monitoring, including consistent follow-up, troubleshooting, and feedback to both patients and physicians, achieved good CPAP compliance rates (≥4 hours per night) of greater than 80% over

6 months.[30] In contrast, close follow-up has not been consistently shown to improve compliance, but is worth doing.[31] Even more effective is to establish adherence and compliance patterns early in treatment initiation, which can help to resolve problems in a timely manner and is essential in the effort to establish a pattern of treatment adherence and good compliance.[21] Intervention early in therapy may improve the patient's early response to CPAP therapy and increase the likelihood that the patient will become a regular and compliant user, thereby enhancing clinical outcome.

Remote continuous positive airway pressure monitoring and fine-tuning

Remote monitoring of health status is one of the objectives of telemedicine.[32–34] It allows clinicians to remotely download previously recorded data.[35–39] Patients can also transmit data on a daily basis into a database (eg, the Encore Anywhere database, Philips; ResTraxx database, ResMed), where data extraction takes place. Next, the data can be analyzed against a set of preestablished criteria or filters. The data set can be scanned for multiple criteria and compared with thresholds for adherence and compliance, trends, AHI, periodic breathing, occurrence of central apneas, and mask leaks.[40] Automatically triggered clinical actions can then be scheduled. An additional goal of such a platform is to proactively identify and address issues that can negatively influence CPAP adherence and compliance. By providing patient data early in the course of CPAP treatment, it is thought that this technology will be extremely useful in improving compliance and acceptance of the device in patients with sleep apnea.[27,35,36,38,40–43] All that is needed is a personal computer, an Internet connection, and the proprietary software. Detailed reports can be generated to show usage information and then forwarded electronically to referral laboratories or physicians without generating additional paperwork. A modem connected to a CPAP unit in the patient's home automatically dials into the server each evening. The compliance server analyzes the data and notifies the physician of any patients with poor CPAP usage. Patient confidentiality is secured through a password and login-protected system that provides protection for the patients' information. Such systems provide accurate, thorough, and advanced information to clinicians and ensure that each patient is receiving the maximum benefit from CPAP therapy. Wireless applications have become available that transmit adherence and compliance data to a central server on a daily base, eliminating the need for data cards, home telephone lines, and frequent patient visits. Clinicians can check their patients at a glance with physician summary reports. Color-coding allows the caregiver to easily identify patients who require attention. Remote setting changes are available to fine-tune therapy and optimize patient management. Historical data can be searched at any time to retrieve data that were not transmitted via the monitoring schedule. As a provider extender, telemedicine support for patients initiating CPAP therapy may allow greater practice efficiency while maintaining quality of care. Roles, expectations, and responsibilities of providers involved in the delivery of such services should be defined and communicated, including those at originating sites and distant sites.[44] The assumptions that parties may have in such encounters and roles should be explicitly documented. In general, the standards for supervision should follow the same general guidelines as those for technicians, respiratory care practitioners, and nurses working with physicians in the live setting. All providers involved have to review their facilities' and institutions' bylaws and human resource documents. Moreover, relevant regulatory documents related to the provision of care are to be followed, and organizations and providers are to ensure that such care is consistent with policies regarding scope of practice and state licensing laws of all involved parties.[44] However, it is questionable whether service providers could be allowed to fine-tune CPAP settings independently, because changing treatment regimens has been the privilege and responsibility of physicians for centuries. To overcome this problem, physicians must be available by telephone to provide assistance and direction if needed. Telemedicine could be readily used to augment general supervision, and asynchronous methods could be used.[44] However, in some countries, CPAP fitting and troubleshooting are not eligible for reimbursement when performed via telemedicine by respiratory therapists and sleep technologists.[44] Nevertheless, study results suggest that the use of telemonitored CPAP compliance and efficacy data seems to be as good as standard care in its effect on compliance rates and outcomes in new CPAP users.[38] Stepnowsky and colleagues[38] showed that a telemonitored clinical care group had a compliance rate of 4.1 hours per night after 2 month, which represents a 46% increase in compliance compared with the mean compliance level of the standard clinical care group (2.8 hours per night). There were some concerns regarding the potential loss of data through wireless transmission. However, the loss was negligible and, once the wireless unit was properly connected, data from previous nights stored on the flow generator device could be retransmitted and obtained wirelessly. Anttalainen and colleagues[45] compared a group of wireless telemonitored CPAP users with a usual-care group, after CPAP titration. They found equal CPAP compliance and residual AHI at 1-year follow-up. Median nursing time was 39 minutes in the telemonitored group and shorter than the 58 minutes per patient in the usual-care group.

Challenges for therapy monitoring

Telemedicine monitoring of sleep apnea therapy is currently limited to CPAP and related ventilator support devices. However, alternative treatment modalities are becoming available. One such option is mandibular advancement devices, which are used to optimize upper airway patency by forcing the mandible into a forward position. It has been shown that these devices can be objectively monitored by in-built thermosensors, with wireless transmission of adherence and compliance data.[46] Also, the data from CPAP devices have to be incorporated with the data regarding the physical status of the patients into the e-Health sleep record. At a later stage, other aspects of digital technology will most likely be incorporated. Among them, integration of relevant health-related data collected from everyday apparel, wearable sensors, and household appliances, and increased interactivity between patients and health care providers, will improve the anticipation and thus, it is hoped, the prevention of the worsening of medical disease states based on validated algorithms.

PATIENT COUNSELING, THERAPY REINFORCEMENT

The use of telemedicine, defined as the use of information and communication technology to deliver health care at a distance, can have a substantial impact on health care use, strengthen the sleep professional–patient interaction, and enhance self-management skills.[47] It has the ability to quickly collect, transmit, and incorporate data, making it a swift and viable means of communication between patients and their providers.[48] These features have a significant potential for the management of patients with OSA, particularly for education and counseling, optimizing CPAP adherence and close monitoring of effective compliance. This type of intervention also has the added potential benefit of fostering patient empowerment. Patients who take ownership, who are involved in their own care, and who possess the knowledge and skills to manage their disease are more likely to comply with lifestyle modifications and treatment regimens, which in turn improves clinical outcomes.[49]

Patient Counseling and Personalized Feedback (Video and Teleconferencing)

Video and telephone contacts provide both direct and indirect benefits to patients. Direct benefits include decreased waiting time and increased physician availability. Indirect benefits include avoidance of barriers to in-person visits, such as the cost and time associated with travel or missed work.[2] Video visits could accommodate chronic routine follow-up appointments. Patient-specific data, such as diaries for insomnia and CPAP machine downloads for OSA, could be reviewed at such visits, as could routine challenges with equipment or medications.[2] A concern could be that the doctor might need to perform some physical examination. However, in sleep medicine it may be that stable patients could be adequately assessed without performing a physical examination that requires the physician to be present in the same room. In addition, certain elements of the examination, such as weight or blood pressure measurement, could be performed at home or by the family physician. In a series of 90 patients with OSA, 56 were seen by a physician at the sleep center and 34 by videoconference. Satisfaction did not differ between the groups.[1]

Promotion and Reinforcement of Patients' Adherence and Compliance

Maximizing adherence and compliance is one of the most important challenges sleep experts face. Telemedicine has been used in various studies to promote and reinforce CPAP treatment.[50–53] In most of them, a cognitive behavioral intervention was applied by telephone,[27,35,41,54,55] the Internet,[35,55] and videoconference.[1,36,56]

Telephone
DeMolles and colleagues[41] used a daily computer-based telephone system to monitor patients' self-reported compliance behavior and provided automated counseling through a structured dialogue. The impact of the intervention was not significant compared with standard care. However, the findings suggest that concurrent education and reinforcement during the initial and early treatment period are effective countermeasures to patient-reported attenuated compliance. Sparrow and colleagues[42] applied an automated telemedicine intervention system, based on an algorithmic interactive voice response system designed to improve CPAP adherence and compliance. The system monitors CPAP-related symptoms and

patients' self-reported behavior and provides feedback and counseling through a structured dialogue to promote CPAP usage. The monitor uses digitized human speech to speak to the patients and the patients communicate via the touch-tone keypad of their telephones. Each call began with an assessment of the self-reported duration and frequency of CPAP usage during the past week, followed by one of several motivational counseling modules. If participants reported excessive side effects or OSA symptoms, the system then recommended the patients to contact their physicians to discuss the problems. The computer system called the patients if they did not make a call at the expected times. Routine printed reports were sent to the participants' physicians biweekly during the first month and the month thereafter. This telemedicine approach resulted in a median CPAP usage that was 0.9 hours per night (at 6 months) and 2.0 hours per night (at 12 months) higher than that of an attention control group.[42] Chervin and colleagues[37] performed a randomized controlled trial (RCT) among 33 patients of 2 interventions to improve compliance: one group received weekly telephone calls to uncover any problems and encourage use, a second group received written information about OSA and the importance of CPAP adherence, and a third group served as a control group. Intervention improved CPAP compliance and the effect was especially strong when intervention occurred during the first month of CPAP treatment. Isetta and colleagues[57] found in a series of 50 consecutive patients with OSA that most of them were satisfied with the teleconsultation method, and 66% agreed that the teleconsultation could replace more than half of their CPAP follow-up visits. In addition, Coma-Del-Corral and colleagues[3] found that the level of good CPAP compliance was 85% at 6 months in patients attending the sleep center for a face-to-face meeting, and 75% in the teleconsultation arm.

Sedhaoui and colleagues[58] performed an RCT in 379 patients with OSA, comparing standard support completed or not within 3 months of coaching sessions, based on telephone-based counseling by competent staff. Sixty-five percent of the patients in the standard group showed a compliance rate of greater than 3 hours per night, versus 75% for the coached group. The mean CPAP usage was 26 minutes longer in the coached group versus the standard group.

Internet
Taylor and colleagues[35] used computers to provide daily Internet-based informational support and feedback for problems experienced during CPAP

usage. Questions related to CPAP use, hours of sleep, and quality of sleep were sent to the participants via a computer. The patients' responses were monitored by the sleep medicine practitioner, and the patient telephoned if deemed necessary. There were no significant differences between the telemedicine intervention and standard-care group at 30 days in patient functional status and satisfaction with CPAP. This intervention only provided self-reported data to the health care provider, whereas objective compliance and detailed physiologic information may have been more useful in effectively troubleshooting problems and may have improved CPAP compliance.[35,56,59] Furthermore, in an RCT, Fox and colleagues[55] showed improved CPAP compliance with a Web-based telemedicine monitoring system. An autoCPAP machine transmitted physiologic data (residual AHI, air leak, compliance) daily to a Web site that could be reviewed. In case problems were identified from data from the Web site, patients were contacted by telephone as necessary. After 3 months, the mean compliance rate was significantly greater in the telemedicine arm (191 min/d), compared with the standard arm (105 min/d). In contrast, 67 minutes of technician time were spent on the patients in the telemedicine arm compared with the standard approach. In addition, Kuna and colleagues[60] found in an RCT that providing patients with daily Web-based access to their positive airway pressure (PAP) usage improves compliance (4.7 ± 3.3 hours in the usual-care group, 5.9 ± 2.5 hours and 6.3 ± 2.5 hours in the Web access groups with and without financial incentive, respectively). Inclusion of a financial incentive in the first week had no additive effect in improving compliance. These findings are consistent with a similar study evaluating the effect on compliance when an interactive Web site providing PAP data to both patients and providers is used.[61]

Video

Smith and colleagues[36] tested a teleconferencing approach in which a nurse visually assessed mask fit and patients' CPAP procedures and provided counseling and reinforcement to patients who were trying CPAP again after an initial 3-month period of poor compliance. Although the patient education materials supplied during the initial period did not affect adherence rates, the nurse teleconferencing sessions during the second trial period substantially improved the adherence of the intervention group (9 of 10 patients vs 4 of 9 in the placebo intervention group), suggesting that intensity of one-on-one counseling and feedback by a care provider is a relevant variable.[36] Isetta and colleagues[57] performed an RCT in which 20

patients with OSA received standard face-to-face training, whereas another 20 received the training via videoconference. Patients showed comparable knowledge about OSA and CPAP therapy, and performance of practical skills was also similar between the two groups. In another study of the same group in 139 patients with OSA, similar levels of CPAP compliance, and improved daytime sleepiness, quality of life, side effects, and degree of satisfaction, were found in a telemedicine-based CPAP follow-up strategy (televisits via video conference based on Skype, e-mail, Web tool support) compared with face-to-face management.[62] Note that the telemedicine group made more extra visits than the face-to-face group, but most of them were non–OSA related.

Integration of Questionnaires, Rating Scales, and Diaries

Questionnaires, rating scales, and diaries can be useful for tracking short-term and long-term results, provided that baseline information is collected. Subsequent data can then be used to monitor symptomatic improvement. Among others, the Functional Outcomes of Sleep Questionnaire (FOSQ) is a popular and well-validated, self-reporting measurement to assess disease-specific health-related quality of life, based on multiple activities of daily living.[63] The FOSQ consists of 32 questions and is available with selected Philips (Murryville, PA) CPAP machines. Data can be remotely downloaded or can be completed or uploaded on a Web-based platform, and can be integrated in the electronic patient record. For patients with comorbid insomnia, telemedicine also provides opportunities to exchange and automatically process sleep diaries and smartphone applications of sleep-wake data, and follow online programs related to cognitive behavior therapy (CBT).[64–66] In this way, the insomnia field can probably be transitioned from evaluating more basic, noninteractive online programs to personalized, interactive online programs. For example, Espie and colleagues[65] used a virtual therapist to help deliver a Web-based CBT-i (CBT for insomnia) program. Such approaches may have more important roles in managing insomnia in the future. Apart from insomnia, it has been shown that the CBT approach is also effective in the context of OSA to improve CPAP adherence.[67] In cases of inadequate sleep hygiene, platforms can be programmed with automated messages to encourage behavioral change, without direct interaction with the sleep provider.[68,69] Clinician and patient satisfaction can be assessed using questionnaires that include visual analog scales and open-ended questions. Patients can be asked to rate their likelihood of continuing to use CPAP, their concern about being monitored, and their overall satisfaction with care. The CPAP self-efficacy scale is a 5-item self-report scale that was developed by Stepnowsky and colleagues.[70] The list of opportunities is almost unlimited. Online platforms will facilitate the movement from disease-based care into patient-based medicine. Such asynchronous tools may provide important diagnostic and therapeutic information. The information from these tools should be easily accessible to sleep providers.[44]

BARRIERS IN THE IMPLEMENTATION OF TELEMEDICINE

Telemedicine aligns with the shift in national focus from technology being used in isolation to technology being the means to both expand the reach of health care and to integrate health care services across patients and organizations. Its adoption has been hampered by a multitude of barriers.

Receptiveness and Willingness of Health Care Providers and Patients

At present, expansion of telemedicine into all aspects of sleep disorder management is limited by the willingness of physicians, patients, and health care organizations to accept telemedicine as an alternative to in-office care.[44] The settings from which patients and physicians originate may influence the perception or acceptance of telemedicine.[1] Croteau and colleagues[71] showed that physicians in urban areas tend to be unwilling to dedicate time to learning how to use new telemedicine equipment. However, if the technology is easy to use, the correlation between ease and implementation is positive. In a study of rural communities, Campbell and colleagues[72] found that physicians are more likely to adopt telemedicine technology if they perceive an increased capability of telemedicine to accommodate the constant advance of technology. In both rural and urban areas, perceived usefulness had the most significant impact on the decision by health care providers to adopt telemedicine. As long as telemedicine can be proved to be a useful tool for health care, the willingness of physicians to use telemedicine technology remains positive. Nevertheless, clinicians' feedback should be further assessed and their involvement promoted as main factor in guaranteeing a successful telemedicine implementation.[73,74] In general, research indicates that telemedicine has been well received by patients with OSA,[1,36] as well as by patients with other medical conditions.[75,76] The greatest advantages of telemedicine that

have been identified are more convenience and decreased travel burden.

Privacy Concerns and Confidentiality

Systems need to be developed to protect patient privacy when CPAP adherence and compliance data reports are reviewed and maintained on servers. A significant current problem in the monitoring of CPAP performance is the ability to track patients with the location data that are transmitted. This ability would violate the right for privacy for the patients being treated. Also, a service provider who monitors not only the usage time but also the flow pattern can provide a diagnosis of the reoccurring sleep apnea as well; for example, it may be caused by a worsening of the disease over time. The patient could be alerted to contact the sleep center, or the applied CPAP pressure could be adjusted remotely. Legal issues may arise, because this is comparable with a medical intervention, such as changing a medication dosage, and such an approach is not allowed in all health care systems.[44] Also, integration of the telemonitored data in the patient sleep record by the home care provider is limited by privacy issues. In France, all these privacy concerns have now led the courts to conclude that there are no legal grounds to allow telemonitoring. Therefore, a robust level of information security for transmission, storage, and access of the data and at the platform in which the data reside is mandatory to implement telemedicine acceptably. This security encompasses strong authentication, data encryption (for both live and stored information), nonrepudiation services, audit logs, a common security policy, and controlled contracts between partners.

The American Academy of Sleep Medicine (AASM) also explicitly describes the following requirements: muting availability; passphrase requirement to access device on which patient data are stored; inactivity timeout function requiring reauthentication with timeout not exceeding 15 minutes; protected health information and confidential data only stored on secure data storage locations; provider knowledge on how patient data are stored and ability to answer patient questions regarding storage of protected health information; access granted only to authorized users; data streamed directly to storage to avoid accidental or unauthorized file sharing.[44] All these requirements are based on American Telemedicine Association guidelines.[77] To encounter security requirements, different data (interchange) standards have been developed.[78] These standards include the primary clinical messaging format standards (eg, the Health Level Seven

[HL7] series) for clinical data messaging; Digital Imaging and Communications in Medicine for medical images; National Council for Prescription Drug Programs script for retail pharmacy messaging; Institute of Electrical and Electronics Engineers (IEEE) standards for medical devices; and Logical Observation Identifiers, Names, and Codes for reporting of laboratory results.[78] Encryption algorithms have been developed for the encryption of electronic data, like the Data Encryption Standard (DES), but the DES was shown to be insecure, because the algorithm was broken in 1993.[79] In addition, the Needham-Schroeder protocol was proved to be insecure more than a decade after its publication.[80,81] More up-to-date encryption standards are the Advanced Encryption Standard (AES), DES-X, GDES, and Triple DES standards, which have been shown to be secure.[82] Alternatives for the DES standard are several replacement algorithms (RC5, Blowfish, IDEA, NewDES, SAFER, CAST5, FEAL, GOST 28147–89, RC6, Serpent, MARS, and Twofish, among many others) with higher security and faster operation.[82,83] For image transfer, specific algorithms have been developed, like the Joint Watermarking-Encryption, which offers confidentiality, integrity, authenticity, and traceability functionalities,[84] and newer algorithms that combine traditional image encryption and image hiding with chaos theory, with improved processing.[85] Nonrepudiation implies that a person cannot deny responsibility for a certain transaction. This principle is important to maintain in audits because a person implicated by an audit should not be able to repudiate responsibility.[79,86,87] Data-access standards for electronic health records (EHRs) are also increasingly being implemented, such as the Fast Health Interoperability Resources, and the Substitutable Medical Applications Reusable Technologies (SMART) Health IT apps interface.[88] From the patient perspective, patient-powered networks are asking for easy download and exchange of their EHR data. Some (unsuccessful) technologies for this purpose were the Consolidated Clinical Document Architecture and the Blue Button.[89] The requirement for certified EHR technologies to provide an application programming interface will enable patients to get access to their EHR data in a timely fashion.[88] Legal liability can be avoided by providing policies and standards for health care providers to observe, like the Health Insurance Portability and Accountability Act (HIPAA) and HL7, which are the standard for encrypting communications and storing medical data in the United States and the United Kingdom.[90–92] Nonrepudiation is necessary to comply with HIPAA, and thus needs to be addressed by all telemedicine systems targeted toward the United States.[87] Also, clear contingency plans are required in the event of loss of communications.[90,91] In addition, controlled contracts between partners are recommended. Such measures are feasible between hospital organizations, and hence for physician-physician contacts, but raise concerns over the ability to develop secure patient-to-physician (or vice versa) data transfer. By only transmitting data relevant to the problem in question, using storing and transmission methods where confidentiality and security are guaranteed, and obtaining informed consent from the patient are ways in which these concerns can be minimized.

Financial Barriers

Although telematic transmission of CPAP adherence and compliance data is the future, a major problem with wireless systems is having the additional resources to retrieve the data,[44] and to cover the costs for providers' services, transmission modules, home installation, licensing fees, telephone charges, security, and additional work by the sleep professionals.[93] These costs should be anticipated by the health care authorities before introducing these technologies. Moreover, despite the evident potential of telemedicine-based interventions, the precise benefits, risks, and costs of this method to deliver health care remain unclear.[94] In a systematic review, telemedicine and telecare services were found to be no more cost-effective than standard health care strategies.[95] In one sleep medicine study, the cost of the interventions, including material costs, was lower than the same number of face-to-face visits,[36] whereas another study reported lower total costs because of savings on transport and less lost productivity (indirect costs).[62] Therefore, a telemedicine-based approach could be especially advantageous if applied to the working population and to residents in medically underserved areas. However, it is important to target and customize these interventions to patients who are most likely to benefit from them. Ultimately, clinicians should also carefully select the appropriate outcomes that telemedicine strategies seek to effect.[96] For example, telemedicine encompasses expanded patient access to quality sleep health care.[97–99] Moreover, protocols need to be developed that describe the roles, expectations, and responsibilities of health care providers, hospitals, physicians, and patients involved in the delivery of sleep telemedicine, because it is not clear when, how, and who should monitor the wireless transmissions. In addition, long-term studies with cost-effectiveness analyses are needed.

Technological Barriers

There are other barriers to incorporating wireless transmission systems routinely in clinical practice. If hospitals make use of different CPAP brands, they will be urged to switch to a single brand in order to control the telemedicine costs. The lack of standardization also precludes interoperability with existing electronic patient records, and data profiles are not standardized between the different providers. Moreover, current electronic patient records are not configured for this type of data management. In addition, there is also the potential for network complications when using a telecommunications network, latency, as well as disconnection. This concern is legitimate, because the potential for complications is a reality.[100] A general concern for telemedicine application includes the lack of reliable Internet access outside of large cities and inadequate bandwidth for high-resolution images or videoconferencing.[101]

Future Platforms

In the older platforms, the organization and management of data were based on a centralized server operating through a call center, with several inherent financial and legal aspects between hospitals and providers.[51] With low-cost miniature integrated circuits now available, new devices have been developed that enable a decentralized communications architecture, whereas the patient's home no longer has to be equipped with any telecommunications infrastructure. Also, smartphone applications are now checked for their diagnostic value, in addition to just monitoring sleep behavior. These developments are rarely validated against medical standards and the diagnostic value is unknown. However, because they allow the transmission of data to the cloud, or even a personal Web page, this is another area in sleep telemedicine that is being realized.[102] However, tracking of patients may also be an issue when using SIM (Subscriber Identity Module) cards, which allow tracking through the wireless transmission cell structure. When the user changes locations, it stores the Location Area Identity number to the SIM and sends it back to the operator network with its new location.[103] Security here is also an issue, particularly when SIM cards use the DES, which is, despite its age, still used by some operators. Cards using the more recent AES or Triple DES standards are secure.[104] Nevertheless, at the moment, these smartphone applications are gadgets in the framework of quantifying an individual, but are not medical supportive tools.[105] It is expected that a full combination of biomedical sensors and mobile phones will also help to incorporate telemedicine into routine practice. However, in a

group of 107 high-cardiovascular-risk patients with OSA, telemonitoring of self-measured home blood pressure, physical activity, and CPAP compliance based on smartphone intervention failed to improve adherence or blood pressure. The investigators speculated that it is possible that telemedicine could be perceived as an additional burden associated with the self-management of blood pressure and CPAP.[106]

Quality Concerns

As recommended by the AASM, clinical standards for telemedicine services should mirror those of live office visits, including all aspects of diagnosis and treatment decisions as would be reasonably expected in office-based encounters.[44] Inherently, physical examination is not possible as it is performed in a face-to-face visit, but is not critical in a sleep medicine setting. Therefore, clinical judgment is mainly based on anamnesis and detailed metrics and analytics. Resources should be made available to reimburse these facilities in a manner competitive or comparable with traditional in-person visits and this will make it feasible to promote a care model in which the different parties involved collaborate and interact, resulting in a better value of health care delivery in a coordinated fashion. Consequently, this also means that appropriate technical standards have to be upheld through the complete telemedicine care delivery process. Therefore, quality assurance processes have to be introduced as well, to ensure the optimal level of patient outcomes, process measures, and user experience. Quality improvement based on data management and quality processing should also be recognized and financially appreciated. Such programs should encompass process measures, patient-centered outcomes, overall provider experience and satisfaction, technical ease, and encryption of communications and storage. Strict application of the highest professional and ethical standards is required, with the aim of improving overall patient access, quality, and value of care. Such an approach benefits from financial transparency throughout the process.[44]

Legal Concerns

Apart from patient privacy, confidentiality, and security concerns, other legal obstacles could arise that focus on the licensure of physicians. It is a universal requirement that physicians practicing within a country must be licensed in that country, whereas in telemedicine, physicians deliver medical treatment across state lines and, possibly, international borders.

Furthermore, the legalities surrounding virtual medical services can sometimes be inconsistent and vague, and can increase liability concerns. Some countries do not allow controlled substances (eg, sedative hypnotics) to be prescribed to patients whom the provider has not seen in a face-to-face encounter. Also, as discussed earlier, data protection and data security are the number 1 issue in any telemedicine application. The EU Directives on the Processing of Personal Data and the Protection of Privacy in the Electronic Communication Sector describe several specific requirements relating to confidentiality and security that telemedicine services have to meet in order to safeguard individuals' rights.[107–109]

If such security can be guaranteed, telemedicine can easily be performed, because any form of communication that does not relate to an identified or identifiable natural person is not subject to the multitude of data protection laws.[107,109] Other European legal achievements related to e-Health are the E-Commerce Directive, the Medical Device Directive, and the Directive on Distance Contracting. These directives are not adopted especially for e-Health applications, but are indirectly important. For store-and-forward encounters that may use digital images of patients for the purpose of rendering a diagnosis or medical opinion, without the presence of the patient, this has been proved feasible for some specialties, like radiology (teleradiology), pathology (telepathology), and dermatology (teledermatology).[110,111] Sleep electroencephalography and polysomnography can also have the interpretation performed remotely.[44] However, in telemedicine with more complex patient/physician encounters using electronic communication and electronic patient records with personally identifiable data, this will be a less achievable goal. Nevertheless, the confidentiality of telemedicine is affected by the inherent risk of third parties intercepting the communication. For example, if a confidential communication is disclosed to a third party, it is not deemed to be confidential, and therefore the physician-patient privilege does not apply.[100] In France, the concept of telemedicine was formalized in the 2009 Hospital, Patients, Health Territories national law and the 2010 decree through which it was applied.[112] Since then, doubts have remained, and, less than 5 years later, sleep telemedicine and remote CPAP compliance monitoring were put on hold, because of privacy concerns. Cloud applications are now being used in some ambitious health care applications, drawing together huge amounts of data from disparately located computers, which implies data sharing across jurisdictions and the sharing of responsibilities by a range of different data controllers.[113] This process could be said to be opening Pandora's Box.

SUMMARY

Various methods are available to assess adherence and compliance with nasal CPAP at home. Objective data can be obtained by either downloads from the memory card of the CPAP device or by direct interrogation of CPAP devices that do not have memory cards. Telemedicine applications can be useful to monitor and motivate patients on a large scale. There are emerging mechanisms for supporting virtual visits and remote monitoring if they can be shown to be financially competitive. Inclusion of sham telemedicine control arms might determine whether increased adherence might have been caused by the perception of monitoring by the patients, or by the more prompt institution of clinical interventions. As this new frontier is explored, it is of paramount importance to be aware of how to use this technology safely, and within the health care system's current legal confines. In addition, careful telemedicine management will provide a more seamless communication flow, to the benefit of medical providers, the global health care system, and ultimately for patients.

REFERENCES

1. Parikh R, Touvelle MN, Wang H, et al. Sleep telemedicine: patient satisfaction and treatment adherence. Telemed J E Health 2011;17(8):609–14.
2. Kelly JM, Schwamm LH, Bianchi MT. Sleep telemedicine: a survey study of patient preferences. ISRN Neurol 2012;2012:135329, 1–6.
3. Coma-Del-Corral MJ, Alonso-Alvarez ML, Allende M, et al. Reliability of telemedicine in the diagnosis and treatment of sleep apnea Syndrome. Telemed J E Health 2013;19(1):7–12.
4. Pelletier-Fleury N, Lanoé JL, Philippe C, et al. Economic studies and 'technical' evaluation of telemedicine: the case of telemonitored polysomnography. Health Policy 1999;49:179–94.
5. Gagnadoux F, Pelletier-Fleury N, Philippe C, et al. Home unattended vs hospital telemonitored polysomnography in suspected obstructive sleep apnea syndrome: a randomized crossover trial. Chest 2002;121(3):753–8.
6. Kristo DA, Eliasson AH, Poropatich RK, et al. Telemedicine in the sleep laboratory: feasibility and economic advantages of polysomnograms transferred online. Telemed J E Health 2001;7:219–24.
7. Kayyali HA, Weimer S, Frederick C, et al. Remotely attended home monitoring of sleep disorders. Telemed J E Health 2008;14:371–4.

8. Bruyneel M, Sanida C, Art G, et al. Sleep efficiency during sleep studies: results of a prospective study comparing home-based and in-hospital based polysomnography. J Sleep Res 2011;20:201–6.

9. Bruyneel M, Van den Broecke S, Libert W, et al. Real-time attended home-polysomnography with telematic data transmission. Int J Med Inform 2013;82(8):696–701.

10. Pelletier-Fleury N, Gagnadoux F, Philippe C, et al. A cost-minimization study of telemedicine. Int J Technol Assess Health Care 2001;17(4):604–11.

11. Masa JF, Corral J, Pereira R, et al. Effectiveness of home respiratory polygraphy for the diagnosis of sleep apnoea and hypopnoea syndrome. Thorax 2011;66:567–73.

12. Fields BG, Behari PP, McCloskey S, et al. Remote ambulatory management of veterans with obstructive sleep apnea. Sleep 2016;39(3):501–9.

13. Seo J, Choi J, Choi B, et al. The development of a nonintrusive home-based physiologic signal measurement system. Telemed J E Health 2005;11:487–95.

14. Choi JM, Choi BH, Seo JW, et al. A system for ubiquitous health monitoring in the bedroom via a Bluetooth network and wireless LAN. Engineering in Medicine and Biology Society 2004. EMBC 2004, conference proceedings. 26th Annual International Conference of the IEEE. Chicago, IL, August 26–30, 2014. p. 3362–5.

15. Böhning N, Zucchini W, Hörstmeier O, et al. Sensitivity and specificity of telemedicine-based long-term pulse-oximetry in comparison with cardiorespiratory polygraphy and polysomnography in patients with obstructive sleep apnoea syndrome. J Telemed Telecare 2011;17:15–9.

16. Boehning N, Blau A, Kujumdshieva B, et al. Preliminary results from a telemedicine referral network for early diagnosis of sleep apnoea in sleep laboratories. J Telemed Telecare 2009;15(4):203–7.

17. Dellaca R, Montserrat JM, Govoni L, et al. Telemetric CPAP titration at home in patients with sleep apnea-hypopnea syndrome. Sleep Med 2011;12:153–7.

18. Collard PH, Pieters TH, Aubert G, et al. Compliance with nasal CPAP in obstructive sleep apnea patients. Sleep Med Rev 1997;1(1):33–44.

19. Engleman HM, Wild MR. Improving CPAP use by patients with the sleep apnea/hypopnea syndrome. Sleep Med Rev 2003;7(1):81–99.

20. Pepin JL, Krieger J, Rodenstein D, et al. Effective compliance during the first 3 months of continuous positive airway pressure: a European prospective study of 121 patients. Am J Respir Crit Care Med 1999;160(4):1124–9.

21. Weaver TE, Kribbs NB, Pack AI, et al. Night to night variability in CPAP use over first three months of treatment. Sleep 1997;20:278–83.

22. Kribbs NB, Pack AI, Kline LR, et al. Objective measurement of patterns of nasal CPAP use by patients with obstructive sleep apnea. Am Rev Respir Dis 1993;147:887–95.

23. Weaver TE, Maislin G, Dinges DF, et al. Relationship between hours of CPAP use and achieving normal levels of sleepiness and daily functioning. Sleep 2007;30(6):711–9.

24. Weaver TE. Predicting adherence to continuous positive airway pressure – the role of patient perception. J Clin Sleep Med 2005;1(4):354–6.

25. Noseda A, Jann E, Hoffmann G, et al. Compliance with nasal continuous positive airway pressure assessed with a pressure monitor: pattern of use and influence of sleep habits. Respir Med 2000;94:76–81.

26. Schwab RJ, Badr SM, Epstein LJ, et al. An official American Thoracic Society Statement: continuous positive airway pressure adherence tracking systems. The optimal monitoring strategies and outcome measures in adults. Am J Respir Crit Care Med 2013;188(5):613–20.

27. Lankford DA. Wireless CPAP patient monitoring: accuracy study. Telemed J E Health 2004;10(2):162–9.

28. Gugger M. Comparison of ResMed AutoSet (version 3.03) with polysomnography in the diagnosis of the sleep apnoea/hypopnoea syndrome. Eur Respir J 1997;10(3):587–91.

29. Barnes M, Houston D, Worsnop CJ, et al. A randomized controlled trial of continuous positive airway pressure in mild obstructive sleep apnea. Am J Respir Crit Care Med 2002;165:773–80.

30. Sin DD, Mayers I, Man GC, et al. Long-term compliance rates to continuous positive airway pressure in obstructive sleep apnea. Chest 2002;121:430–5.

31. Rodenstein DO. How to improve compliance to nasal continuous positive airway pressure in sleep apnoea syndrome. Monaldi Arch Chest Dis 1998;53(5):586–8.

32. Friedman RH, Kazis LE, Jette A, et al. A telecommunications system for monitoring and counseling patients with hypertension: impact on medication adherence and blood pressure control. Am J Hypertens 1996;9:285–92.

33. Smith CE, Cha JJ, Kleinbeck SV, et al. Feasibility of in-home telehealth for conducting nursing research. Clin Nurs Res 2002;11:220–33.

34. Smith CE, Mayer LS, Perkins SB, et al. Caregiver learning needs and reactions to managing home mechanical ventilation. Heart Lung 1994;23:157–63.

35. Taylor Y, Eliasson A, Andrada T, et al. The role of telemedicine in CPAP compliance for patients with obstructive sleep apnea syndrome. Sleep Breath 2006;10(3):132–8.

36. Smith CE, Dauz ER, Clements F, et al. Telehealth services to improve nonadherence: a placebo-controlled study. Telemed J E Health 2006;12(3):289–96.

37. Chervin RD, Theut S, Bassetti C, et al. Compliance with nasal CPAP can be improved by simple interventions. Sleep 1997;20:284–9.

38. Stepnowsky CJ Jr, Palau JJ, Marler MR, et al. Pilot randomized trial of the effect of wireless telemonitoring on compliance and treatment efficacy in obstructive sleep apnea. J Med Internet Res 2007;9(2):e14.

39. Cooper CB. Respiratory applications of telemedicine. Thorax 2009;64:189–91.

40. Isetta V, Thiebaut G, Navajas D, et al. E-telemed 2013: Proceedings Fifth International Conference on e-Health, Telemedicine and Social Medicine Nice, France, February 24–March 1, 2013. p. 156–61.

41. DeMolles DA, Sparrow D, Gottlieb DJ, et al. A pilot trial of a telecommunications system in sleep apnea management. Med Care 2004;42:764–9.

42. Sparrow D, Aloia M, Demolles DA, et al. A telemedicine intervention to improve adherence to continuous positive airway pressure: a randomised controlled trial. Thorax 2010;65:1061–6.

43. Fraysse JL, Delavillemarque N, Gasparutto B, et al. Home telemonitoring of CPAP: a feasibility study. Rev Mal Respir 2012;29:60–3.

44. Singh J, Badr MS, Diebert W, et al. American Academy of Sleep Medicine (AASM) position paper for the use of telemedicine for the diagnosis and treatment of sleep disorders. J Clin Sleep Med 2015; 11(10):1187–98.

45. Anttalainen U, Melkko S, Hakko S, et al. Telemonitoring of CPAP therapy may save nursing time. Sleep Breath 2016. [Epub ahead of print].

46. Dieltjens M, Braem M, Vroegop A, et al. Objectively measured vs. self-reported compliance during oral appliance therapy for sleep-disordered breathing. Chest 2013;144(5):1495–502.

47. Paré G, Jaana M, Sicotte C. Systematic review of home telemonitoring for chronic diseases: the evidence base. J Am Med Inform Assoc 2007;14: 269–77.

48. Seibert PS, Valerio J, DeHaas CA. The concomitant relationship shared by sleep disturbances and type 2 diabetes: developing telemedicine as a viable treatment option. J Diabetes Sci Technol 2013;7(6):1607–15.

49. Gellis ZD, Kenaley B, McGinty J, et al. Outcomes of a telehealth intervention for homebound older adults with heart or chronic respiratory failure: a randomized controlled trial. Gerontologist 2012;52(4):541–52.

50. Verbraecken J. Compliance monitoring in CPAP therapy. ERS buyers' guide. 2011; 77–87.

51. Farré R. The future of telemedicine in the management of sleep-related respiratory disorders. Arch Bronconeumol 2009;45(3):109–10.

52. Meurice JC. Improving compliance to CPAP in sleep apnea syndrome: from coaching to telemedicine. Rev Mal Respir 2012;29:7–10.

53. Kwiatkowska M, Ayas N. Can telemedicine improve CPAP adherence? Thorax 2010;65(12):1035–6.

54. Leseux L, Rossin N, Sedkaoui K, et al. Education of patients with sleep apnea syndrome: feasibility of a phone coaching procedure. Phone coaching and SAS. Rev Mal Respir 2012;29(1):40–6.

55. Fox N, Hirsch-Allen AJ, Goodfellow E, et al. The impact of telemedicine monitoring system on positive airway pressure adherence in patients with obstructive sleep apnea: a randomized controlled trial. Sleep 2012;35(4):477–81.

56. Spaulding R, Stevens D, Velasquez SE. Experience with telehealth for sleep monitoring and sleep laboratory management. J Telemed Telecare 2011; 17(7):346–9.

57. Isetta V, Leon C, Torres M, et al. Telemedicine-based approach for obstructive sleep apnea management: building evidence. Interact J Med Res 2014;3:e6.

58. Sedkaoui K, Leseux L, Pontier S, et al. Efficiency of a phone coaching program on adherence to continuous positive airway pressure in sleep apnea hypopnea syndrome: a randomized trial. BMC Pulm Med 2015;15:102.

59. Kwiatkowska M, Idzikowski A, Matthews L. Telehealth-based framework for supporting the treatment of obstructive sleep apnea. Stud Health Technol Inform 2009;143:478–83.

60. Kuna ST, Shuttleworth D, Chi L, et al. Web-based access to positive airway pressure usage with or without an initial financial incentive improves treatment use in patients with obstructive sleep apnea. Sleep 2015;38(8):1229–36.

61. Stepnowsky C, Edwards C, Zamora T, et al. Patient perspective on use of an interactive website for sleep apnea. Int J Telemed Appl 2013;2013: 239382.

62. Isetta V, Negrin MA, Monasterio C, et al. A Bayesian cost-effectiveness analysis of a telemedicine-based strategy for the management of sleep apnoea: a multicentre randomised controlled trial. Thorax 2015;70:1054–61.

63. Weaver TE, Laizner AM, Evans LK, et al. An instrument to measure functional status outcomes for disorders of excessive sleepiness. Sleep 1997; 20(10):835–43.

64. Ritterband LM, Thorndike FP, Gonder-Frederick LA, et al. Efficacy of an internet-based behavioural intervention for adults with insomnia. Arch Gen Psychiatry 2009;66(7):692–8.

65. Espie CA, Kyle SD, Williams C, et al. A randomized, placebo-controlled trial of online cognitive behavioral therapy for chronic insomnia disorder delivered via an automated media-rich web application. Sleep 2012;35:769–81.

66. Anderson KN, Goldsmith P, Gardiner A. A pilot evaluation of an online cognitive behavioral therapy for

insomnia disorder – targeted screening and interactive Web design lead to improved sleep in a community population. Nat Sci Sleep 2014;6:43–9.

67. Richards D, Bartlett DJ, Wong K, et al. Increased adherence to CPAP with a group cognitive behavioral treatment intervention: a randomized trial. Sleep 2007;30(5):635–40.

68. Mastin DF, Bryson J, Corwyn R. Assessment of sleep hygiene using the sleep hygiene index. J Behav Med 2006;29(3):223–7.

69. Stepnowsky C, Sarmiento KF, Amdur A. Weaving the internet of sleep: the future of patient-centric collaborative sleep health management using web-based platforms. Sleep 2015;38(8):1157–8.

70. Stepnowsky CJ Jr, Marler MR, Ancoli-Israel S. Determinants of nasal CPAP compliance. Sleep Med 2002;3:239–47.

71. Croteau AM, Vieru D. Telemedicine adoption by different groups of physicians. Proceedings of the 35th Hawaii International Conference on System Sciences (HICSS '02). Hawaii, January 7–10, 2002. p. 151–9.

72. Campbell JD, Harris KD, Hodge R. Introducing telemedicine technology to rural physicians and settings. J Fam Pract 2001;50:419–24.

73. Demiris G, Oliver DR, Fleming DA, et al. Hospice staff attitudes towards telehospice. Am J Hosp Palliat Care 2004;21(5):343–7.

74. Prescher S, Deckwart O, Winkler S, et al. Telemedical care: feasibility and perception of the patients and physicians: a survey-based acceptance analysis of the Telemedical Interventional Monitoring in Heart Failure (TIM-HF) trial. Eur J Prev Cardiol 2013;20(2 Suppl):18–24.

75. Harrison R, Macfarlane A, Murray E, et al. Patient's perceptions of joint teleconsultations: a qualitative evaluation. Health Expect 2006;9:81–90.

76. Azad N, Amos S, Milne K, et al. Telemedicine in a rural memory disorder clinic-remote management of patients with dementia. Can Geriatr J 2012;15:96–100.

77. Gough F, Budhrani S, Cohn E, et al. Practice guidelines for live, on demand primary and urgent care. Telemed J E Health 2015;21:233–41.

78. Aspden P, Corrigan JM, Wolcott J, et al. Health care data standards. In: Committee on Data Standards for Patient Safety, editor. Patient safety: achieving a new standard for care. Washington: The National Academies Press; 2004. p. 127–68. Chapter 4.

79. Makris L, Argiriou N, Strintzis MG. Network access and data security design for telemedicine applications. Presented at: 2nd IEEE Symposium on Computers and Communications. Alexandria, Egypt, July 1–3, 1997.

80. Needham RM, Schroeder MD. Using encryption for authentication in large networks of computers. Comm ACM 1978;21(12):993–9.

81. Lowe G. An attack on the Needham-Schroeder public key authentication protocol. Inform Process Lett 1995;56(3):131–6.

82. Data Encryption Standard – Wikipedia. Accessed August 3, 2016.

83. Alfandi O, Bochem A, Kellner A, et al. Secure and authenticated data communication in wireless sensor networks. Sensors (Basel) 2015;15:19560–82.

84. Bouslimi D, Coatrieux G, Cozic M, et al. A joint encryption/watermarking system for verifying the reliability of medical images. IEEE Trans Inf Technol Biomed 2012;16:891–9.

85. Dai Y, Wang H, Zhou Z, et al. Research on medical image encryption in telemedicine systems. Technol Health Care 2016;24:S435–42.

86. Garg V, Brewer J. Telemedicine security: a systematic review. J Diabetes Sci Technol 2011;5(3):768–77.

87. Ferrante FE. Evolving telemedicine/ehealth technology. Telemed J E Health 2005;11(3):370–83.

88. Mandl KD, Kohane IS. Time for a patient-driven health information economy? N Engl J Med 2016;374(3):205–8.

89. D'Amore JD, Mandel JC, Kreda DA, et al. Are meaningful use stage 2 certified EHRs ready for interoperability? Findings from the SMART C-CDA Collaborative. J Am Med Inform Assoc 2014;21:1060–8.

90. HIPAA documentation. Available at: www.hipaadvisory.com. Accessed August 3, 2016.

91. Atchinson BK, Fox DM. The politics of the health insurance portability and accountability act. Health Aff 1997;16(3):146–50.

92. Available at: http://www.hl7.org. Accessed August 3, 2016.

93. Zia S, Fields BG. Sleep telemedicine: an emerging field's latest frontier. Chest 2016;149(6):1556–65.

94. Isetta V, Ruiz M, Farré R, et al. Supporting patients receiving CPAP treatment: the role of training and telemedicine. ERS Monogr 2015;67:280–92.

95. Mistry H. Systematic review of studies of the cost-effectiveness of telemedicine and telecare. Changes in the economic evidence over twenty years. J Telemed Telecare 2012;18:1–6.

96. Wilson SR, Cram P. Another sobering result for home telehealth – and where we might go next. Arch Intern Med 2012;172(10):779–80.

97. Hirshkowitz M, Sharafkhaneh A. A telemedicine program for diagnosis and management of sleep-disordered breathing: the fast-track for sleep apnea tele-sleep program. Semin Respir Crit Care Med 2014;35(5):560–70.

98. Watson NF. Expanding patient access to quality sleep health care through telemedicine. J Clin Sleep Med 2016;12(2):155–6.

99. Baig MM, Antonescu-Turcu A, Ratarasarn K. Impact of sleep telemedicine protocol in management of

sleep apnea: a 5-year VA experience. Telemed J E Health 2016;22(5):458–62.

100. Clark PA, Capuzzi K, Harrison J. Telemedicine: medical, legal and ethical perspectives. Med Sci Monit 2010;16(12):RA261–72.

101. World Health Organization. Telemedicine: opportunities and developments in member states: report on the second global survey on eHealth. Geneva (Switzerland): WHO; 2010.

102. Penzel T, Glos M, Garcia C, et al. Sleep medicine integrates telemedicine methods in diagnosis and treatment. Proceedings International Society on Biotelemetry. 21st Symposium. Leuven (Belgium), May 22–24, 2016.

103. Saad ZA. Next generation mobile communications ecosystem. Hoboken (NJ): John Wiley & Sons; 2011. p. 306.

104. SR Labs. Rooting SIM cards. Available at: https://srlabs.de/rooting-sim-cards. Accessed August 3, 2016.

105. Penzel T. Sleep quality challenges and opportunities. IEEE EMB Pulse 2016.

106. Mendelson M, Vivodtzev I, Tamisier R, et al. CPAP treatment supported by telemedicine does not improve blood pressure in high cardiovascular risk OSA patients: a randomized, controlled trial. Sleep 2014;37(11):1863–70.

107. European Parliament and European Council. Directive 95/46/EC on the protection of individuals with regard to the processing of personal data and the free movement of such data. Brussels (Belgium): European Parliament and European Council; 1995.

108. European Commission. Telemedicine for the benefit of patients, healthcare systems and society. Commission Staff Working paper EC (2009) 943 final. Brussels, Belgium, 2009.

109. European Parliament and the Council of the European Union. Directive 2002/58/EC concerning the processing of personal data and the protection of privacy in the electronic communications sector. Brussels (Belgium): European Parliament and the Council of the European Union; 2002.

110. Ruotsalainen P. Privacy and security in teleradiology. Eur J Radiol 2010;73:31–5.

111. Dierks C. Legal aspects of telepathology. Anal Cell Pathol 2000;21:97–9.

112. Zannad F, Maugendre P, Audry A, et al. Telemedicine: what framework, what levels of proof, implementation rules. Therapie 2014;69(4):339–54.

113. Callens S, Cierkens K. Legal aspects of E-HEALTH. Stud Health Technol Inform 2008; 141:47–56.

Sleep Applications to Assess Sleep Quality

Ingo Fietze, MD, PhD

KEYWORDS

- Sleep disturbance • Smartphone applications • Polysomnography • Actimeters • Insomnia

KEY POINTS

- Applications in smartphones offer the promised possibility of detection of sleep.
- From the author's own experience, one can also conclude that sleep applications are approximately as good as polysomnography in detection of sleep time and sleep efficiency, similar to the conventional wearable actimeters.
- In the future, sleep applications will help to further enhance awareness of sleep health and to distinguish those who actually poorly and only briefly sleep from those who suffer more likely from paradox insomnia.

In the age of telecommunications, smartphones, and telemedicine, it is only logical that the topics of healthy and disturbed sleep have come under examination. Furthermore, there are runaway developments in applications for smartphones on the Internet. Although these applications have heightened public perception for the topic of sleep, which is a good sign, they have on the other hand not attained the level of scientific validation.

In this context, standards in the diagnosis of healthy and disturbed sleep have become established and are continuously being modified.[1] The technological standard here is cardiorespiratory polysomnography, as well as simple polysomnography, for study of sleep profiles. Polysomnography measures the sleep stages and latency, sleep efficiency, total sleep time (TST), activity, body position, and wake time during sleep, including arousal. Until now, standards have not been developed in this context for sleep stage transition, body turning, dynamics of changes in sleep stages, the length of the nonrapid eye movement (NREM)-rapid eye movement (REM) cycle, the sleep spindle count, and many other parameters.

The time has now arrived to validate these data with respect to their significance, and to stay abreast of current and future technological progress. Such validation is essential to maintain justified applicability of polysomnography in the future. On the other hand, there will be consumer sleep technologies (CSTs) that will provide data that come very close to those obtained from polysomnography (PSG) sleep data. CST developments include mobile device platforms (ie, sleep apps), wearable platforms, embedded platforms, desktop and website platforms, as well as accessory appliance platforms.[2] Sleep apps, definitely among these developments, are still far from satisfying the PSG standard, as will be described.

SLEEP APPLICATIONS IN SMARTPHONES

Stradling and colleagues[3] very well may have created the predecessor of the first application for sleep research, before smartphones as we know them came onto the market. They developed a combination of a mobile video camera with oximetry to record sleep apnea at home. Our applications in smartphones today promise the possibility of sleep detection. These applications are based on accelerometry, and in certain cases with support of additional sensor systems and/or parameters such as light sensors, on microphones to detect day/night data, phone usage, and sleep diaries. Essentially, conventional accelerometry, such as for fitness trackers and clinical actigraphs, is based

Center of Sleep Medicine, Charité – Universitätsmedizin Berlin, Luisenstr 13, Berlin 10117, Germany
E-mail address: ingo.fietze@charite.de

Sleep Med Clin 11 (2016) 461–468
http://dx.doi.org/10.1016/j.jsmc.2016.08.008
1556-407X/16/© 2016 Elsevier Inc. All rights reserved.

on the principle of 3-axis micromechanical systems (MEMS). The most popular accelerometers use piezoelectric microcrystals or capacitive elements to convert movements into electrical signals.[4]

In contrast, the principle of accelerometry in smartphones is a black box and therefore unknown.

At the same time, however, sleep applications have become extremely popular. In 2014, Sleep Tracker and Alarm Clock were the most downloaded applications on iTunes. This is remarkable when one also considers that in early 2014, the Apple iTunes shop offered around 100,000 health applications and more than 500 applications for sleep monitoring.[2] The best-known sleep applications today include Sleep Cycle, SleepBot, Sleep As Android, Sunriser, and Go to Sleep.[2] **Fig. 1** shows an actual Google Play sleep application search. What should one make of these extensive offerings? How should the consumer decide? Which applications should or can a physician recommend?

In this context, it is helpful to know what these applications can actually do, in comparison to polysomnography, the gold standard. Few investigations have been conducted on these issues. Recently, Bhat and colleagues[5] conducted a polysomnographic study of 20 volunteers (aged 20–57 years) with healthy sleeping habits, in parallel with application of the app Sleep Time (Azumio, Incorporated, Palo Alto, California). There were no correlations in findings between the 2 methods for the following: sleep efficiency, sleep onset latency, or sleep stage percentages for light sleep and deep sleep. The application Sleep Time underestimated light sleep and overestimated deep sleep and sleep latency and achieved very low accuracy in epoch-wise comparison (45.9%). Discrimination between wake and sleep was much better

(85.9%). Sensitivity in detection of sleep is accordingly high (89.9%), but specificity is low (50%).

From the author's experience, one can also conclude that sleep applications are approximately as good as polysomnography in detection of sleep time, similar to the conventional wearable actimeters. Sleep applications, however, like wearable actimeters (**Fig. 2**) cannot distinguish between the stages of sleep or between light und deep sleep, which is, however, suggested by most of the wearable actimeters and most of the applications. These limitations, however, disclose at the same time a particular shortcoming of all available sleep applications: that is, it is not known which algorithms work behind the accelerometric detection offered. Indeed. It is well known that the application of different algorithms for the same data results in different results. Natale and colleagues in 2012[6] applied 3 different actigraphy algorithms to smartphone accelerometer data. The differences between actimetry and smartphone accelerometry depended on the algorithms applied, and the smartphone data were poorer than data from wearable actigraphs. Another interesting finding of this study was that the differences in TST, waking after sleep onset (WASO), and sleep efficiency (SE) increased for TST less than 6 hours, SE below 85%, and WASO greater than 20 minutes. In other words, the poorer the sleep, the less reliable the results from sleep applications. Similar differences could possibly be likewise expected as a function of the specific accelerometer hardware being used in a smartphone. Unfortunately, the hardware components are basically unknown, with information – unlike Domingues 2015 – only rarely published on this aspect. Until now, there have been no studies

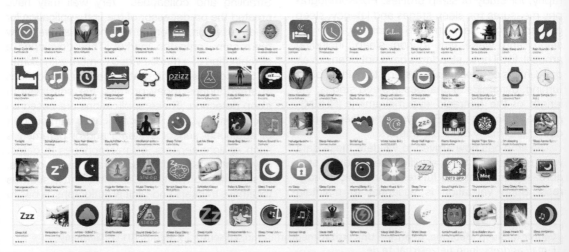

Fig. 1. Extract of the android applications by Google. (Available at: https://play.google.com/store/search?q=sleep%20apps&c=apps&hl=de. Accessed July 8, 2016.)

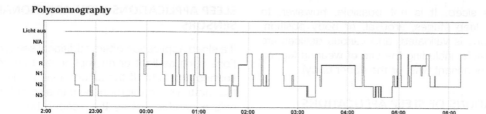

Polysomnography

Stage 1: 37 min (9.2% TST)

Stage 2: 185 min (46.2% TST)

Stage 3: 92 min (23 % TST)

REM sleep: 85.5 min (21.6% TST)

Wake after sleep onset: 69.4 min

Wearable actigraphy

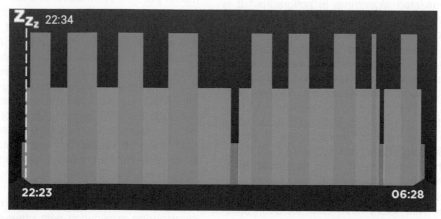

Light sleep: 432 min

Deep Sleep: 229 min

Awake for: 22 min

Fig. 2. Comparison of polysomnography with wearable actigraphy in one volunteer (good sleeper).

that investigate the influence of the hardware on such sleep data quality.

Toon and colleagues in 2015[7] published a further study that compared PSG with a smartphone application. The investigation involved the application MotionX 24/7 in use with children, and revealed underestimation of sleep onset latency (SOL) and WASO, and overestimation of TST and SE.

In 2015, with 27 volunteers between 20 and 59 years of age, Min and colleagues[8] compared the sleep application Toss N Turn, not with PSG, but with an electronic version of the Pittsburgh Sleep Quality Index (PSQI). There were differences in bedtime, sleep duration, and wake time by more than 30 minutes in all 3 parameters.

If, in summary, comparison is made between smartphone applications with wearable actigraphy—which, to be sure, come close to polysomnography, with sensitivity of 78.8% to 99.7%[9]—the data from the applications are poorer.

The choice between clinically graded actigraphy and smartphone accelerometry will be based on technology, price, and reliability. Sleep researchers and sleep physicians, however, can and must exert influence here. Until now, conventional actimetry has established its significance in investigations of sleep–wake rhythm disorders, hypersomnia, and insomnia, especially among athletes and shift workers. If light-out times and light-on times are known, either by documentation in a diary or by a light sensor in an actimeter, it is possible to estimate satisfactorily the effective sleep time, WASO, and SOL.[10] The movement index also allows good conclusions on restful and restless sleep. It is not possible, however, to detect sleep stages, arousal, or body position. Actigraphy is validated, and various devices are comparable, including the site of wearing (eg, on the nondominant wrist or the upper body).

LIMITATIONS OF SLEEP APPLICATIONS

Use of an application in a smartphone, in contrast, depends on the location of the smartphone on the mattress, its characteristics, and—as Bianchi notes[11]—the presence of a partner. As a result, it is not possible to apply the standards of conventional actigraphy to smartphone applications. Another obstacle for validity check of smartphone accelerometric data is the fact that raw data are not generated that can be confirmed and processed. The algorithms are closed in comparison to well-validated algorithms in actigraphs.[4] It is not known, for example, how any of these applications calculate sleep duration.

Sleep applications also present an additional, major restriction to wearables and fitness trackers; they cannot evaluate relevant data during daytime waking. Although actimeters are also not very effective in this context (sensitivity: 48.5%–79.8%), they represent, in addition to a sleep log, the only instrument for assessment of resting and/or sleeping phases during the day.

A further restriction of sleep applications involves their use by senior citizens, people with sleep disorders, and patients with major health problems. Actimeters have also not been satisfactorily validated for these people.[12] For those with sleep disorders, for example, there is overestimation of their SOL. The fact that sleep applications (eg, Sleep Time) also suffer from these restrictions intensifies the problem of false-positive results.[4]

At this point we must consider additional functions, supplementary sensors, and the possible future employment of sleep applications. Many sleep applications today also promise optimal waking during the light sleep phase – a function that appeals, for example, to nurses.[13] But there has been no documented evidence of the benefits of such optimal waking, nor has there been validation of detection of the light sleep phase – and, in turn, of the fact that waking in fact takes place during light sleep.[3] Would it not be better, for example, to actually take advantage of the brief period that a person may have for sleep in bed, than to get up 30 minutes earlier? The probability of being woken from deep sleep early in the morning, with sleep inertia, is very slight – and does not justify a trend toward increasingly early waking among, for example, our young people.

SLEEP APPLICATIONS WITH ADDITIONAL SENSORS

If a sleep application offers additional sensor functions such as light or microphones, it can detect sounds and light. If the smartphone is placed on the mattress, its microphone can also detect signals generated not by the sleeper, but by his or her partner. Another example of difficulty is with people who have PLM syndrome. If the smartphone is positioned such that it can record these movements, then it allows false conclusions of poor sleep. Periodic limb movements without arousal, however, do not disturb sleep architecture, with the result that false negative results occur here as well. Even upon assumption of smartphone sleep application accuracy of 99% for TST, this still produces 1000 false measurements per 100,000 measurements.[14]

One solution would be to especially install additional sensors at the subjects' feet, to detect or rule out periodic leg movement.[15] At least from the clinical standpoint, the combination of a sleep application and one or several wearable electroencephalography (EEG)/electrooculography (EOG) and EMG sensors offers a promising approach. Although the ZEO system (ZEO Inc) has not survived[2] – despite the fact that the sleep tracking software was validated[16] – this technology will most probably be applied increasingly, at least in sleep medicine. Currently, the company Somnomedics (Randersacker, Germany) has marketed a new and expanded system. A combination of a smartphone application with other sensors such as the EMG for the PLM syndrome, or a body-position sensor for sleepwalking, would also be feasible.

In 2014, Garde and colleagues[17] presented a screening tool for sleep-disordered breathing in children, with application of phone oximetry. The benefits include ease of operation, convenience, and the possibility of measuring several times. Noncontact measuring systems are similar in this respect: for example, unobtrusive ballistocardiography.[18] A piezoelectric film sensor under the mattress topper sends heart rate, respiratory variation, activity, and sleep-stage data to the web server. Such systems enable long-term measurements, both for diagnostic purposes as well as for therapy monitoring.

SNORING APPLICATIONS

Although audio detection of snoring by smartphones has not yet been validated,[19] there is also no measurement standard in polysomnography – even in 2016 – for this frequent symptom.

Arnardottir and colleagues[20] have evidenced that recording by a microphone is clearly more nearly valid than by nasal-pressure measurement or other methods. As a result, snoring applications definitely offer prospects of success. In 2015, Camacho and colleagues[21] found 126 snoring applications in the Apple iTunes application store. Four authors have investigated 13 of these applications at home tests with one patient. In addition, these applications were compared with polysomnography for 2 patients. These 13 applications satisfied inclusion and exclusion criteria, which included the requirements for recording of data, graphical analysis, playback, and the like. Apart from the problem of the threshold (which can be variously set) and background noise (which can falsify any result), the authors concluded the following: (1) Select smartphone snoring applications can be useful for recording and playing back snorting sounds; (2) The most critical application feature is the ability to graphically display nocturnal events, with a zooming function for second-by-second analysis; (3) The applications demonstrate excellent positive predictive value for application snoring detection (93.3%–96%); and (4) More user studies are required to enhance the relevance of these applications.

DIAGNOSTIC AND THERAPEUTIC SLEEP APPLICATIONS

Increasingly, applications are also being marketed that allow diagnosis or tentative diagnosis on the basis of questionnaires. Applications are also available that support therapy for sleep disturbance. Zluga and colleagues[22] have countered the problem of nonsupervised completion of questionnaires with the Rolling Score Concept. Here, a specific time schedule has been added to each question. This concept, applied in cases of the STOP-Bang questionnaire, the Berlin questionnaire, and the PSQI, allows results with only 7% deviation of scores.

If a smartphone is positioned on the body, detection of respiration and circulation is also feasible – or possible with an additional sensor. This would enable detection of respiratory disorders or arrhythmia, as well as sleep data derived from heart rate.[23] Therapeutic sleep applications tested in studies include applications that determine, support, or conduct cognitive behavioral therapy for insomnia.

In a pilot trial, Koffel and colleagues[24] tested a CBT-I coach (cognitive behavioral treatment for insomnia) and evidenced its feasibility and benefits. In a randomized, placebo-controlled trial with 3 arms – CBT, imagery relief therapy (IRT: placebo), and treatment as usual (TAU) – Espie and colleagues[25] verified that web-based CBT is effective.

Kuhn and colleagues[26] reached similar conclusions for insomnia patients, as did Min and colleagues[27] in cancer patients with insomnia. These promising approaches should be quickly integrated into clinical practice, since the number of patients continues to rise – but is not matched to the same degree by increased offerings for CBT, primarily owing to great human-resources and time expenditures.

OUTLOOK

Although this reservation also applies to clinical actigraphs, there is 1 major difference; clinical actigraphs are applied only on a small scale, since sleep physicians are never confronted with 100,000 potential patients per day. If, however, the use of these sleep applications continues to increase, and if attention to the dangers of poor sleep continues, then there will be more and more persons who come to with self-diagnosis based on self-gathered data.[28] Van Bulck[29] describes how mercurial business with applications is, how fast they come and go. But the number of applications will continue to rise: from sales of 2.5 million in 2014 to an estimated 26 mission in 2017.[30]

How can one use sleep applications in the future? To begin, one must realize that the attention of the general public has been focused on normal sleep parameters such as sleep efficiency, TST, and SOL. If a healthy LOS can be state today,[31] then there should also be the possibility simply to measure sleep length with validity, as is currently possible with blood pressure and peak flow. If sleep applications are presently developing toward this goal, then scientific support for this development should be provided, a conclusion that also represents an appeal to the developers of software and hardware for smartphones. Indeed, lack of validation studies for most of the sleep applications is a pressing concern.

In addition to sleep duration, sleep efficiency is a highly important parameter. This ratio of sleeping and waking during the period from light out to light on is a parameter that can be well represented and effectively determined and that can as well be measured with good, approximate validity by actigraphy. A proportion of greater than 85% means satisfactory sleep; between 70% and 85% signifies impaired sleep, and less than 70% indicates poor sleep. Future memory studies—in contrast to those until now in which primarily sleep duration has been varied—should investigate whether sleep efficiency in these classifications represents a good parameter for cognitive performance. This would enable future users of sleep applications also to apply the results for their daily scheduling and for performance management.

Today it is known that impaired sleep over the long run, and/or short nights, not only compromise quality of life, but also influence life expectancy.[32] As a result, in the future physicians will be forced to examine more and more patients who have sensitive or impaired sleep. Validated sleep applications would be well suited for this purpose. This requires, however, that these applications be tested not only on healthy sleepers, as until now, but also on people with sleep disorders. Present sleep applications are not suited for continuous measurements, day and night, or over several days, which are necessary for shift workers, athletes, and workers with irregular working schedules.[33,34] Supplementing a sleep application with an additional actimeter sensor, which would automatically transmit the data to the cell phone, would enable employment of these sleep applications for these patient groups also.

A smartphone can also effectively detect bruxism; studies comparing with PSG are currently underway in the author's facilities. Special speech technologies will also enable detection of sleep talking, and camera techniques can offer the recording of periodic limb or body movements.[15]

The PowerNap Wecker is an entirely different form of a sleep application. The concept involves holding a smartphone in the napper's hands, with finger contact on the surface of the phone. When the user falls into a power nap, the pressure on the surface diminishes, and the contact fails, which causes the phone to sound an alarm. The author and colleagues conducted a study on this effect; the study, however, was broken off and not published. The author and colleagues unfortunately learned that the finger contact diminished so quickly—after only a few seconds or minutes—that a refreshing nap was not possible. This application is an example that an initially good idea, even one that can be successfully marketed, cannot necessarily be proven effective in scientific reality.

In the future, sleep applications will help to further enhance awareness of sleep health and to distinguish those who actually poorly and only briefly sleep from those who suffer more likely from paradox insomnia. Additionally, they would likely help in saving the considerable expense of diagnostic measures in a sleep laboratory. In other fields of sleep medicine (eg, detection of sleep apnea), they can definitively help to guide the right patients sooner to effective therapy[35–37] and to

afford enhanced monitoring of continuous positive airway pressure therapy.[36] It would also prove beneficial to implement therapy supervision of other disorders such as insomnia and restless legs syndrome. Already today, sleep applications for cognitive behavior treatment are helping to substitute for shortages in human resources.[38]

Sleep applications should find their proper place when embedded in a system of telemedicine and telehealth, a development that has not yet taken place.[38] A prerequisite here is establishment of standards for detection and evaluation, similar to current attempts for portable sleep apnea monitors used in telemedicine.[39]

Legal liability and governmental regulation of consumer health technologies, including those related to sleep and sleep disorders, are developing fields that are currently in their infancy. As legislative reform pends, more extensive randomized trials are needed to elucidate impact on patient outcomes, cost, and health care system accessibility.

If there is success in enabling sleep application developers and sleep specialists to closely collaborate, then the medical field will be well on its way to establishing smartphone application detection of healthy and disturbed sleep on a validated foundation and to provide the status for this topic in telehealth that obesity, fitness, and the like enjoy already today. Imagine a future in which sleep information and technology are fully integrated into the home and into the consumer's lifestyle. Consumers themselves will then be able to monitor their own sleep, actively measure sleep conditions and their outcomes, prevent sleep disorders, recognize such impairment in good time, and consult a sleep specialist at the optimal point in time.

REFERENCES

1. Berry RB, Brooks R, Gamaldo CE, et al. Vaughn BV for the American Academy of Sleep Medicine. The AASM manual for the scoring of sleep and asociated events: rules, terminology and technical specifications, version 2.3. Darien (IL): American Academy of Sleep Medicine; 2016.

2. Ko PR, Kientz JA, Choe EK, et al. Consumer sleep technologies: a review of the landscape. J Clin Sleep Med 2015;11(12):1455–61.

3. Stradling JR, Thomas G, Belcher R. Analysis of overnight sleep patterns by automatic detection of movement on video recordings. J Amb Monitor 1988;1(3):217–32.

4. Kolla BP, Mansukhani S, Mansukhani MP. Consumer sleep tracking devices: a review of mechanisms, validity and utility. Expert Rev Med Devices 2016; 13(5):497–506.

5. Bhat S, Ferraris A, Gupta D, et al. Is there a clinical role for smartphone sleep Apps? Comparison of sleep cycle detection by a smartphone application to polysomnography. J Clin Sleep Med 2015;11(7):709–15.

6. Natale V, Drejak M, Erbacci A, et al. Monitoring sleep with a smart-phone accelerometer. Sleep Biol Rhythms 2012;10(4):287–92.

7. Toon E, Davey MJ, Hollis SL, et al. Comparison of Commercial Wrist-Based and Smartphone Accelerometers, Actigraphy, and PSG in a Clinical Cohort of Children and Adolescents. J Clin Sleep Med 2016;12(3):343–50.

8. Min J-K, Doryab A, Wiese J, et al. Toss 'n' turn: smartphone as sleep and sleep quality detector. In: Jones M, Palanque P, Schmidt A, et al, editors. Proceedings of the SIGCHI conference on human factors in computing systems. Toronto: Association for Computing Machinery; 2014. p. 477–86.

9. Tryon WW. Nocturnal activity and sleep assessment. Clin Psychol Rev 1996;16(3):197–213.

10. Morgenthaler T, Alessi C, Friedman L, et al. Standards of Practice Committee; American Academy of Sleep Medicine Practice parameters for the use of actigraphy in the assessment of sleep and sleep disorders: an update for 2007. Sleep 2007;30(4):519–29.

11. Bianchi MT. Consumer sleep apps: when it comes to the big picture, it's all about the frame. J Clin Sleep Med 2015;11(7):695–6.

12. Sadeh A. The role and validity of actigraphy in sleep medicine: an update. Sleep Med Rev 2011;15(4): 259–67.

13. Haidrani L. Sleep Cycle alarm clock app. Nurs Stand 2016;30(29):31.

14. Behar J, Roebuck A, Domingo JS, et al. A review of current sleep screening applications for smartphones. Physiol Meas 2013;34:R29–46.

15. Madhushri P, Ahmed B, Penzel T, et al. Periodic leg movement (PLM) monitoring using a distributed body sensor network. Conf Proc IEEE Eng Med Biol Soc 2015;2015:1837–40.

16. Shambroom JR, Fábregas SE, Johnstone J. Validation of an automated wireless system to monitor sleep in healthy adults. J Sleep Res 2012;21:221–30.

17. Garde A, Dehkordi P, Karlen W, et al. Development of a screening tool for sleep disordered breathing in children using the phone Oximeter™. PLoS One 2014;9(11):e112959. http://dx.doi.org/10.1371/journal.pone.0112959. eCollection 2014.

18. Paalasmaa J, Waris M, Toivonen H, et al. Unobtrusive online monitoring of sleep at home. Conf Proc IEEE Eng Med Biol Soc 2012;2012:3784–8.

19. Stippig A, Hübers U, Emerich M. Apps in sleep medicine. Sleep Breath 2015;19(1):411–7.

20. Arnardottir ES, Isleifsson B, Agustsson JS, et al. How to measure snoring? A comparison of the microphone, cannula and piezoelectric sensor. J Sleep Res 2016;25(2):158–68.

21. Camacho M, Robertson M, Abdullatif J, et al. Smartphone apps for snoring. J Laryngol Otol 2015; 129(10):974–9.

22. Zluga C, Modre-Osprian R, Kastner P, et al. Continual Screening of Patients Using mHealth: The Rolling Score Concept Applied to Sleep Medicine. Studies in Health Technology and Informatics. Volume 223: Health Informatics Meets eHealth. p. 237–44.

23. Penzel T, Kantelhardt JW, Grote L, et al. Comparison of detrended fluctuation analysis and spectral analysis for heart rate variability in sleep and sleep apnea. IEEE Trans Biomed Eng 2003;50(10):1143–51.

24. Koffel E, Kuhn E, Petsoulis N, et al. A randomized controlled pilot study of CBT-I Coach: Feasibility, acceptability, and potential impact of a mobile phone application for patients in cognitive behavioral therapy for insomnia. Health Informatics J 2016. [Epub ahead of print].

25. Espie CA, Kyle SD, Williams C, et al. A randomized, placebo-controlled trial of online cognitive behavioral therapy for chronic insomnia disorder delivered via an automated media-rich web application. Sleep 2012;35(6):769–81.

26. Kuhn E, Weiss BJ, Taylor KL, et al. CBT-I Coach: A Description and Clinician Perceptions of a Mobile App for Cognitive Behavioral Therapy for Insomnia. J Clin Sleep Med 2016;12(4):597–606.

27. Min YH, Lee JW, Shin YW, et al. Daily collection of self-reporting sleep disturbance data via a smartphone app in breast cancer patients receiving chemotherapy: a feasibility study. J Med Internet Res 2014;16(5):e135.

28. Topol E. The creative distruction of medicine: how the digital revolution will create better health care. New York: Basic Books; 2012.

29. Van den Bulck J. Sleep apps and the quantified self: blessing or curse? J Sleep Res 2015;24(2):121–3.

30. Reserach2guidance. mHealth app developer economics 2014, the state of the art of mHealth app publishing. Berlin: Research2guidance; 2014.

31. Hirshkowitz M, Whiton K, Albert SM, et al. National Sleep Foundation's updated sleep duration recommendations. Sleep Health 2015;1(4):233–43.

32. Parthasarathy S, Vasquez MM, Halonen M, et al. Persistent insomnia is associated with mortality risk. Am J Med 2015;128(3):268–75.e2.

33. Fietze I, Knoop K, Glos M, et al. Effect of the first night shift period on sleep in young nurse students. Eur J Appl Physiol 2009;107(6):707–14.

34. Fietze I, Strauch J, Holzhausen M, et al. Sleep quality in professional ballet dancers. Chronobiol Int 2009;26(6):1249–62.

35. Baig MM, Antonescu-Turcu A, Ratarasarn K. Impact of sleep telemedicine protocol in management of sleep apnea: a 5-Year VA experience. Telemed J E Health 2016;22(5):458–62.

36. Fox N, Hirsch-Allen AJ, Goodfellow E, et al. The impact of a telemedicine monitoring system on positive airway pressure adherence in patients with obstructive sleep apnea: a randomized controlled trial. Sleep 2012;35(4):477–81.

37. Anttalainen U, Melkko S, Hakko S, et al. Telemonitoring of CPAP therapy may save nursing time. Sleep Breath 2016. [Epub ahead of print].

38. Zia S. Fields BG sleep telemedicine: an emerging field's latest frontier. Chest 2016; 149(6):1556–65.

39. Hirshkowitz M, Sharafkhaneh A. A telemedicine program for diagnosis and management of sleep-disordered breathing: the fast-track for sleep apnea tele-sleep program. Semin Respir Crit Care Med 2014;35(5):560–70.

Sleep Assessment in Large Cohort Studies with High-Resolution Accelerometers

Melanie Zinkhan, PhD[a,*], Jan W. Kantelhardt, PhD[b,c]

KEYWORDS

- Accelerometers • Actigraphy • Sleep-wake differentiation • Periodogram-based sleep detection
- Cohort studies • German National Cohort

KEY POINTS

- Large prospective studies are needed to identify sleep characteristics as possible determinants of personal health.
- Accelerometers can be a practical replacement for polysomnography in large observational studies.
- State-of-the-art accelerometers can estimate population-based average sleep times reasonably, at least for populations without high prevalence of sleep problems.
- Further algorithm development is required, as conventional classification approaches do not exploit major aspects of the acceleration data and work for wrist-worn devices only.
- Accompanying quality assurance procedures are necessary for accelerometer recordings in large cohort studies.

INTRODUCTION: SLEEP AND HEALTH

Insomnia and other sleep disturbances are discussed to be associated with impaired functioning during the day and higher risks for work or traffic accidents.[1–4] Beyond impacts on daytime performance, there is evidence on associations between insomnia, sleep apnea, or general sleep characteristics (such as shortened or prolonged sleep duration) with risk factors for major diseases,[5–9] morbidity,[10–16] and mortality.[15,17–21] However, the explanatory value of many studies on these associations is limited because of restrictions of the underlying study designs, or limitations in methods used for the assessment of the respective exposures. For example, a cross-sectional design, relying on self-reported information on sleep, residual confounding, and measurement artifacts might limit the results.[22–24] Therefore, it is premature to infer causal relationships from the current body of literature. Hence, additional large prospective studies, such as cohort studies, are needed that address sleep characteristics as possible determinants of personal health in more differentiated ways.

Conflict of Interest: None of the authors declared any conflict of interest.

[a] Institute of Medical Epidemiology, Biostatistics and Informatics, Faculty of Medicine, Martin-Luther-University Halle-Wittenberg, Magdeburger Str 8, Halle 06112, Germany; [b] Institute of Physics, Faculty of Natural Sciences II, Martin-Luther-University Halle-Wittenberg, Von-Seckendorff-Platz 1, Halle 06099, Germany; [c] Cardiovascular Physics, Department of Physics, Humboldt-University of Berlin, Robert-Koch-Platz 4, Berlin 10115, Germany
* Corresponding author.
E-mail address: melanie.zinkhan@uk-halle.de

Sleep Med Clin 11 (2016) 469–488
http://dx.doi.org/10.1016/j.jsmc.2016.08.006

ASSESSMENT OF SLEEP IN MEDICINE AND RESEARCH

Cardiorespiratory polysomnography (PSG) has been regarded as the gold standard in sleep medicine since 1968.[25–28] However, the applicability of PSG for the assessment of sleep characteristics in large prospective studies is limited due to its intricacy and costs.[29] Beyond that, PSG may produce first-night effects[30–32] and may lead to a selection bias because not every participant agrees with staying overnight in a sleep laboratory,[12,33] whereas participants might differ systematically from nonparticipants. Additionally, PSG settings might influence sleep depending on individual factors.[34–37] Therefore, conclusions based on PSGs might be limited with regard to sleep under unattended conditions at home.

As an alternative to PSGs, movement-based methods, such as actigraphy (or accelerometry) have been established since 1974.[38–41] They are also used for measuring physical activity and other physiologic signals in ambulatory settings.[42] Advantages of accelerometry over PSG are described as lower costs, higher availability, easy recording of multiple nights, and lower influence on natural sleep.[43–46] Nevertheless, movement-based methods seem to overestimate sleep and to underestimate wakefulness.[43,47,48] Their accuracy varies between different sleep variables[49] and depends on population-specific characteristics, being reduced the more sleep is disturbed.[43,47] In clinical settings, accelerometers are thus recommended only as an adjunct in the evaluation of circadian rhythm disorders, the assessment of sleep patterns in healthy adult populations, and in inpatients with certain suspected sleep disorders, such as delayed sleep phase syndrome or shift work disorder. They are not recommended as diagnostic instruments for routine diagnosis.[50,51]

The validity of movement-based devices also depends on device-specific technical characteristics and the algorithm used for data analysis. Technological progress leads to advanced devices with higher temporal resolution, higher acceleration resolution, and separate recording of all 3 directions (see later in this article), whereas many published and still used algorithms are several years old.[52,53] We refer to **Box 1** for short descriptions of several algorithms published between 1992 and 2013. Most algorithms do not take high resolutions into account or use aggregated data only.[54–57] As an early exception, in 2004, Hedner and colleagues[58] described an algorithm for a single-axis actigraph with a sampling rate of 100 Hz, reporting a reasonable sensitivity and specificity in patients with sleep apnea. For using this algorithm with more recent 3-axis devices, the applicability and validity would have to be tested. In conclusion, there seems to be a lack of algorithms for the deduction of sleep characteristics from recent high-resolution 3-axis accelerometers that are actually used in large observational studies.

SLEEP ASSESSMENT IN POPULATION-BASED STUDIES

This section gives a none-exhaustive overview of some important population-based studies with sleep assessments until 2016. One of the first articles on the frequency of sleep disturbances in a general population was published by Bixler and colleagues[59] in 1979. Since then, many population-based studies have included more or less comprehensive sleep assessments based on self-reported data (questionnaire or interview data).[60–64] Since 1988, objective measurements on sleep also have been applied with a special focus on sleep-related disorders, see **Table 1**. Initially, the focus was on sleep-disordered breathing (SDB),[65–68] whereas most recent cohort studies assess information on sleep as potential exposures or outcomes of interest among many others.[62,69–74]

THE GERMAN NATIONAL COHORT STUDY: A LARGE PROSPECTIVE OBSERVATIONAL STUDY

The German National Cohort (GNC) is an ongoing cohort study with objective measurements on sleep. This prospective observational study has been designed to provide a resource for population-based health and disease research in Germany, with a focus on major chronic diseases; that is, cardiovascular diseases, cancer, diabetes, neurodegenerative/psychiatric diseases, musculoskeletal diseases, respiratory and infectious diseases, and their preclinical stages or functional health impairments.[74] Study centers across Germany aim at including a total of 200,000 subjects (100,000 men, 100,000 women, 20–69 years of age) randomly sampled from the general population during 4 to 5 years since 2014. The overall duration is planned for 25 to 30 years. The baseline assessment includes a personal interview, self-completion questionnaires, medical examinations, samples taken for a bio bank, and an accelerometer (GT3X+; ActiGraph, Pensacola, FL) worn at the hip for 7 days.[74,86] A random subsample of 40,000 participants receives an intensified examination program (see later in this article), and

Box 1
Sleep detection algorithms for accelerometers

Most algorithms are designed for analyzing "counts," which represent the aggregated motion intensity over epochs between 10 and 60 seconds. All algorithms have been developed for accelerometers placed at the patient's wrist of the nondominant arm. All of them calculate, for each epoch, a weighted average (linear combination) of several parameters (with a corresponding number of weight coefficients, **Table 2**) and compare its value with a threshold. A value below the fixed threshold usually indicates "sleep" epochs.

- Cole and colleagues[52] (1992) calculated weighted averages of the activity counts during four 1-minute epochs before and 2 epochs after the current epoch (with epochs overlapping by 10 seconds). The same algorithm was used by de Souza and colleagues[94] (2003).

- Sadeh and colleagues[53] (1994) used a linear model (corresponding to a weighted average) of 4 parameters: (1) the activity counts in a window of 11 minutes centered around the current 1-minute epoch, (2) the number of epochs among these 11 with activity levels between 50 and 100 counts, (3) the standard deviation (SD) of activity counts during the current epoch and the 5 epochs preceding it, and (4) the logarithm of the number of activity counts during the next epoch.

- Gorny and colleagues[95,96] (1996, 1997) classified 30-second epochs according to the sum of activity counts in 9 surrounding epochs; that is, the current epoch and 4 epochs before, as well as 4 epochs after the current epoch. Dick and colleagues[97] (2010) applied the same algorithm to data recorded with the recent SOMNOwatch plus device using a threshold of 28 "units" (no clear definition of "unit" is given).

- Jean-Louis and colleagues[98] (2001) studied 30-second scoring results of an undisclosed algorithm relying on single-axis accelerometer data sampled at 20 Hz with merely 8-bit resolution.

- Hedner and colleagues[58] (2004) suggested the first algorithm for accelerometers recording at 100 Hz, but just on 1 axis. They applied a narrow digital band pass filter (2.0–2.5 Hz) and compared the "energy" in this band with the background movement activity of the patient throughout the night. In this comparison, weighted averages over a sliding window of 5 minutes and patient-specific thresholds were used. In addition, to take apneic events into account, the threshold was locally raised if cyclic variations with periods from 12 to 90 seconds occurred.

- Enomoto and colleagues[56] (2009) ignored accelerations below 0.06 g and calculated weighted averages of the acceleration intensities 4 minutes and 2 minutes before and after as well as during the scored 30-second epoch. This algorithm was also applied to time series of counts in 2-minute epochs by Nakazaki and colleagues[54] (2014), who derived different coefficients for the same linear model.

- Kripke and colleagues[57] (2010) calculated weighted averages of the activity counts in 21 epochs around the current 30-second epoch, but found that epochs more than 1 minute after the current one did not help in improving the classification.

- Galland and colleagues[55] (2012) suggested a rescaling of counts with respect to the whole-night average of epochs with non-zero counts, comparing results for 15-second, 30-second, and 60-second epochs and using the algorithms of Cole and colleagues[52] (1992) and Sadeh and colleagues[53] (1994).

- Wohlfahrt and colleagues[93] (2013) described a periodogram-based sleep detection (PBSD) algorithm relying on 3-axis accelerometer data with high sampling rate (see also main text). Their weighted averages are calculated from 5 parameters that characterize the data's power spectra in epochs of 30 seconds.

30,000 participants take part in a whole-body MRI program.[74,87] Four to 5 years after the baseline assessment, all participants will be invited to a reassessment. Outcomes of interest will be assessed by a combination of active follow-up every 2 to 3 years and record-linkages.[74,88]

Sleep characteristics are assessed by a self-completion questionnaire that is based on the Pittsburgh Sleep Quality Index (PSQI),[89] the Berlin Questionnaire (Berlin-Q),[90] and the German version of the Morningness-Eveningness Questionnaire (D-MEQ).[91,92] Due to the large amount of questions, the questionnaires are not applied in their full versions. Nevertheless, it is possible to get reliable information on the following sleep-related characteristics: subjective sleep quality, sleep latency, sleep duration, sleep efficiency, sleep disturbances (difficulties falling asleep, difficulties maintaining sleep, early morning awakening), daytime sleepiness, sleep-disordered breathing, daytime napping, and circadian preference.

Table 1
Selected cohort studies with objective measurements on different sleep characteristics

Study	Country	Initiation	Age Range, y	Population	n[a]	Sleep Measurement Recordings	Sleep Measurement Scoring
Wisconsin Sleep Cohort Study (WSCS)[65,75]	USA	1988	30–60	Male and female state employees of Wisconsin Oversampling of subjects at high risk of sleep-disordered breathing	1550	Single-night PSG (in laboratory) Channels: EEG, EOG, EMG, ECG, nasal AF, oral AF, tracheal sounds (microphone), thoracic and abdominal respiratory effort, SpO$_2$	Rechtschaffen & Kales[25] 1968
Busselton Sleep Cohort[66,76]	Australia	1990	40–65	Male and female residents of Busselton	400	4-channel sleep apnea home-monitoring device (MESAM IV) Channels: snoring, HR, SpO$_2$, body position	Manual
Penn State Cohort[68,77]	USA	1993	20–100	Male and female residents of southern Pennsylvania Oversampling of subjects at high risk of sleep-disordered breathing	1741	Single-night PSG (in laboratory) Channels: EEG, EOG, EMG, nasal AF, oral AF, thoracic respiratory effort, SpO$_2$	Rechtschaffen & Kales[25] 1968
Sleep Heart Health Study (SHHS)[67]	USA	1995	≥40	Male and female participants of existing cohorts on cardiovascular diseases (Atherosclerosis Risk in Communities Study, Cardiovascular Health Study, Framingham Heart Study, 3 New York Cohorts, Strong Heart Study, 2 Tucson Cohorts) Oversampling of habitual snorers	6424	Single-night in-home PSG Channels: EEG, EOG chin EMG, thoracic and abdominal respiratory effort, nasal-oral thermistry, SpO$_2$, ECG, body position, ambient light level	Rechtschaffen & Kales[25] 1968 Additional SHHS criteria[78]

Study	Country	Age	Year	N	Population	Assessment	Software/Criteria
Study of Osteoporotic Fractures (SOF)[69]	USA	≥65	1986 (sleep since 2002)	3127	Female community-dwelling participants of 4 US areas (Baltimore, Minneapolis, Portland, Monongahela Valley)	≥3 d of wrist actigraphy Sleepwatch-O (aggregated accelerometry data over 1 min, 3 different modes)	Action W2 software, algorithms by Cole et al,[52] 1992 and Jean-Louis et al,[79] 2001
				461	Convenience subsample with PSG	Single-night in-home PSG Channels: EEG, EOG, chin EMG, thoracic and abdominal respiratory effort, nasal-oral thermistry, nasal AF, SpO₂, ECG, body position, leg movements	Rechtschaffen & Kales,[25] 1968
Osteoporotic Fractures in Men (MrOS)[80]	USA	≥65	2003	3135	Male community-dwelling participants of 6 US areas (Birmingham, Minneapolis, Palo Alto, Portland, Monongahela Valley, San Diego)	≥5 d of wrist actigraphy with Sleepwatch-O (aggregated accelerometry data over 1 min, 3 different modes)	Action W2 software, algorithm by Cole et al,[52] 1992 and Jean-Louis et al,[79] 2001
				2862	Subsample with PSG	Single-night in-home PSG Channels: EEG, EOG, chin EMG, thoracic and abdominal respiratory effort, nasal-oral thermistry, nasal AF, SpO₂, ECG, body position, leg movements	SHHS criteria[78]
Heinz Nixdorf Recall Study[71,81]	Germany	45–75	2000 (sleep since 2006)	1604	Male and female residents of 3 cities in the Ruhr area (Essen, Bochum, Mühlheim)	Single-channel screening for sleep-disordered breathing for 1 night with ApneaLink device	ApneaLink scoring software 5.13

(continued on next page)

Table 1
(continued)

Study	Initiation	Country	Age Range, y	Population	n[a]	Sleep Measurement	
						Recordings	Scoring
Study of Health in Pomerania[72]	2002 (sleep since 2008[b])	Germany	20–79	Male and female residents of the Federal State of Mecklenburg/West Pomerania	1266	Single-night PSG (in laboratory) Channels: EEG, EOG, EMG (chin, tibialis), nasal AF, thoracic and abdominal respiratory effort, body position, SpO_2, HR, snoring	AASM 2007 criteria[26]
HypnoLAUS[82]	2003 (sleep since 2009)	Switzerland	49–68	Male and female residents of the city of Lausanne	2121	Single-night in-home PSG, PSG setup according to AASM 2007 recommendations[26]	AASM 2013 criteria[27]
UK Biobank[62,83,84]	2006 (accelerometry since 2009)	United Kingdom	40–69	Male and female residents from UK	103,720	7 d of 3-axial accelerometry at the wrist; recordings were conducted for the measurement of physical activity; sleep scoring possible	No specific concepts for sleep scoring so far

Study	Country	Year	Age	Population	N	Device / recordings	Scoring
LIFE-Adult-Study[73,85]	Germany	2011	18–79	Male and female residents of the city of Leipzig	2767	7 d of 2-axial accelerometry with the multiple sensor SenseWear Pro 3 device; additional recordings: skin temperature, near body ambient temperature, heat flux, galvanic skin response, motion	SenseWear Professional software
German National Cohort Study[74]	Germany	2014 (ongoing)	20–69	Male and female residents of Germany	Up to 160,000; (ongoing)	7 d of 3-axial accelerometry at the hip with ActiGraph GT3X plus; recordings were conducted for the measurement of physical activity; sleep scoring possible	No specific concepts for sleep scoring so far
					Up to 40,000; (ongoing)	24 h of 3-axial accelerometry at the wrist with SOMNOwatch plus device; additional recordings: 1-lead ECG, nasal flow during night	Periodogram-based sleep detection algorithm[93]

Abbreviations: AF, airflow; ECG, electrocardiography; EEG, electroencephalography; EMG, electromyography; EOG, electrooculography; HR, heart rate; SpO₂ oxygen saturation.

a Number of participants with measurements on sleep.
b Sleep measures were performed in SHIP-TREND cohort.

In addition to the questionnaire, 24-hour accelerometry concurrently recorded by the SOMNOwatch plus device (SOMNOmedics, Randersacker, Germany) with a 24-hour electro-cardiogram (ECG) and nocturnal airflow has been established as an objective assessment of sleep characteristics for the intensified examination program of 40,000 participants. Because of their intricacy, applicability, and costs, it is not possible to perform PSG examinations in the sleep laboratory or at home. However, because modern multipurpose devices can record other physiologic signals concurrently with accelerometry, they seem very attractive for large observational studies and future applications also beyond the GNC.

ACCELEROMETRY: PRINCIPLE AND STATE-OF-THE-ART DEVICES

Accelerometers measure the force F on an internal test mass m (or test masses) with respect to a freely falling reference frame. The readout of acceleration $a = -F/m$ is usually quantified in terms of g-force; that is, in fractional multiples of the standard gravitational acceleration $g_0 = 9.81$ m/s^2 on the surface of the earth. The indicated acceleration will be zero if the sensor is in freefall, but not if it is at rest in a gravitational field. Therefore, an accelerometer at rest on the earth will indicate an acceleration of approximately 1g *upward*, as it is accelerated upward compared with freefall. If the accelerometer is moved, it will indicate additional g-force components during the start of the motion (acceleration phase) and during the end of the motion (deceleration phase), but not during a motion at constant velocity. Because force F and

acceleration a are vectors, there are 3 components that can be recorded independently.

State-of-the-art accelerometers record accelerations at sampling rates of approximately 100 Hz (ie, 100 measurements per second) separately for 3 perpendicular directions (usually termed x, y, and z) and can store the data from several days in their internal memory. The g-force values a_x, a_y, and a_z are usually recorded at 12-bit resolution; that is, in steps of $12 \text{ g}/2^{12} = 0.0029 \text{ g} = 2.9$ mg if the range is from +6g to −6g (values for SOMNOwatch plus). Typical noise levels of such sensors are in the range of 10 to 20 mg for the absolute value $a = |a| = \sqrt{a_x^2 + a_y^2 + a_z^2}$. Most accelerometer sensors are micro-electro-mechanical devices, consisting of 2 tiny interwoven bar structures linked by a spring. If the sensor is accelerated, the distance between the fixed bars and the movable bars will change by a few tens of nanometers. The change of the capacitance between the bars is then evaluated by electronic circuits deriving the g-force value. In the device, 3 such sensors are usually mounted perpendicular to each other to measure a_x, a_y, and a_z.

ACCELEROMETRIC TIME SERIES RECORDED DURING SLEEP AND SLEEP SCORING

During sleep, accelerometers attached to a subject's wrist or hip record only weak motion activity for most of the time. This can be seen in **Fig. 1**, where all 3 components are basically flat except for sharp steps associated with nocturnal position changes (roll overs) and a few intermediate wakefulness episodes. We note that the absolute orientation of the accelerometer device with respect to

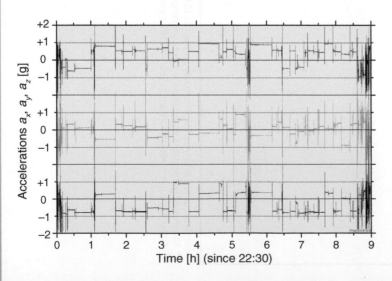

Fig. 1. Components a_x (top), a_y (middle, cyan), and a_z (bottom) of the acceleration vector as measured by an accelerometer (SOMNOwatch plus) attached to a subject's wrist during a typical night (from 22:30 to 07:30) in units of g-force (see text). Position changes lead to step-like behavior, because the direction of the gravitational component changes (besides weak additional acceleration). Only during short episodes of wakefulness (eg, at 04:00 shown at 5.5 hours) the accelerometer records nonsteady behavior.

the vertical direction (gravitational force) can be determined exactly from the g-force values at these plateaus. However, because hardly any structure besides the steps was noticed in accelerometer recordings during sleep, such as those shown in **Fig. 1**, most sleep evaluation algorithms (**Box 1** and **Table 2**) are based on a threshold for the total acceleration strength and score epochs with accelerations below the threshold as sleep. All of these algorithms work in the time domain and consider windows of at least 4.5 minutes' duration. Only quite recently, we have shown that sleep scoring might be improved by taking additional features of the acceleration signals into account, which can be detected by spectral analysis[93] (see later in this article). That algorithm also can be applied to accelerometer data recorded at the hip.

In addition, we would like to note that the recordings of current state-of-the-art accelerometers are not exactly constant during sleep even without position changes. Their high sensitivity allows the detection of very weak motions that are, for example, caused by respiratory activity. This is shown in **Fig. 2**, where a short sequence of the data from **Fig. 1** is presented with mean values subtracted and vertical scale magnified by a factor of nearly 1000. Although the motion caused by respiration is quite close to the g-force resolution and the measurement noise level (note the steps of digitalization and the random fluctuations between neighboring steps in **Fig. 2**), it can be clearly identified in the smoothed signal.

SPECTRA OF ACCELEROMETRIC TIME SERIES ACROSS SLEEP AND WAKE

Recently, we have, probably for the first time, studied spectra (periodograms) of high-resolution accelerometric time series recorded at the wrists and hips of 100 subjects during sleep and wake with simultaneous PSG as part of the preparation of the GNC study.[93] **Fig. 3** shows the average spectra for all episodes of light sleep, deep sleep, and rapid-eye movement (REM) sleep, as well as wakefulness during the night and wakefulness during the day. The oscillation caused by respiration (cf. see **Fig. 2**) can be clearly identified with the peak at 0.2 to 0.3 Hz in the spectra. The frequency of 0.2 to 0.3 Hz translates to a period of 5.0 to 3.3 seconds and corresponds to human respiration during rest with an average frequency of 12 to 18 breaths per minute in adults. Periodic components with integer multiple frequencies of the respiratory base frequency, that is, higher harmonics, also are observed, for example at approximately 0.6 Hz and 0.9 to 1.0 Hz. Another band with an increased intensity is visible at 6 to 10 Hz. This periodic signal, which has different strength in different subjects, has a

Table 2
Comparison of sleep detection algorithms relying on accelerometer recordings

Author	Sampling Interval	Epoch Length	Axes	Number of Tuned Coefficients	Window Backward	Window Forward
Cole et al,[52] 1992	1 min	1 min	1	3	4 min	2 min
Sadeh et al,[53] 1994	1 min	1 min	1	4	5 min	5 min
Gorny et al,[95] 1996	30 s	30 s	1	3	2.25 min	2.25 min
Jean-Louis et al,[98] 2001	0.05 s (20 Hz)	30 s	1	Undisclosed	Undisclosed	Undisclosed
Hedner et al,[58] 2004	0.01 s (100 Hz)	30 s	1	None	2–5 min	2–5 min
Enomoto et al,[56] 2009	30 s	30 s	1	5	4 min	4 min
Kripke et al,[57] 2010	30 s	30 s	1	14	5 min	1 min
Galland et al,[55] 2012	15–60 s	15–60 s	1	3–4	4–5 min	2–5 min
Wohlfahrt et al,[93] 2013	0.0078 s (128 Hz)	30 s	3	5	5 min	0 min

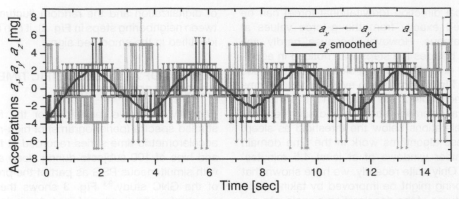

Fig. 2. Components a_x, a_y, and a_z (in units of mg, ie, 10^{-3} g-force) during 15 seconds, while there is no position change. The means (plateau values) have been subtracted for each component. Besides the random sensor noise, one can see an oscillation caused by respiration. The periodicity is clearer for the smoothed curve, where a running average filter (width 2 seconds) has been applied to a_x (*thick red curve*).

broader-frequency spectrum than respiration. We think that these periodicities are caused by physiologic tremor.

Fig. 4 shows color-coded time-resolved spectrograms of wrist acceleration together with the corresponding hypnogram based on PSG. Strong movements (red vertical lines in the spectrogram) occur during wakefulness. In addition, almost every transition from N3 to N2, N1, or wake is associated with body movements. Arm movements or roll overs in bed are typical movements during sleep stage transitions and also lead to high intensities in the spectrograms without a preferred frequency (yellow or red vertical lines, for example at 2 hours, 2 hours 40 minutes, 3 hours 40 minutes, 4 hours 45 minutes, and 5 hours 30 minutes). REM sleep is characterized by a reduced muscle tone and a shallow breathing. This is reflected by low spectral power, see for

example the REM sleep episode at approximately 3.6 to 4.4 hours. However, one observes strong variations among REM episodes within a single subject and among different subjects. High intensities in the frequency band around 0.3 Hz are permanently observed across all sleep stages (horizontal band colored yellow or green). The power is reduced during REM sleep due to the overall low spectral power. Nevertheless, **Fig. 4** suggests that accelerometer data could be used to track approximately the respiratory rate throughout the night, although the device was worn at the wrist.

Comparable spectrograms are obtained for accelerometers worn at the hip; see **Fig. 5** as an example from another healthy subject. The presence of a respiratory peak could also be used to distinguish sleep episodes from periods in which the accelerometer is not worn by the subject.

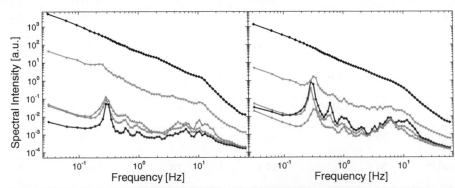

Fig. 3. Periodograms of wrist acceleration (averages of the curves for a_x, a_y, and a_z) for different sleep stages (*light blue: light sleep N1 and N2; dark blue: deep sleep N3; orange: REM sleep*), wake during night (*green*), and wake during day (*black*) for 2 typical healthy subjects from the GNC pretest data. (*Data from* Wohlfahrt P, Kantelhardt JW, Zinkhan M, et al. Transitions in effective scaling behavior of accelerometric time series across sleep and wake. Europhys Lett 2013;103(6):68002.)

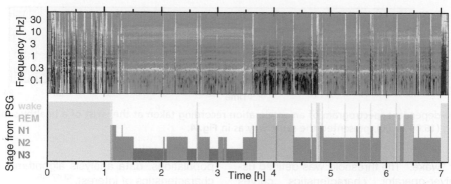

Fig. 4. Time-dependent spectrogram of a nocturnal acceleration recording taken at the wrist of a healthy subject. The periodograms were calculated for each 30-second epoch of the signals using Fast Fourier Transform (FFT), logarithmically wide frequency bins have been applied, and the spectral power is color coded (*red: large power; green: intermediate power; blue: small power*). The subject's sleep stages (hypnogram) based on polysomnography (*green: wake; blue: light sleep; dark blue: deep sleep; orange: REM sleep*) are shown below the spectrograms. (*Data from* Wohlfahrt P, Kantelhardt JW, Zinkhan M, et al. Transitions in effective scaling behavior of accelerometric time series across sleep and wake. Europhys Lett 2013;103(6):68002.)

The latter is illustrated in **Fig. 6**, where all structure is missing from the spectrogram during nearly 1 hour from approximately 20:30 to 21:25. During daytime, much stronger accelerations occur at all frequencies (see **Figs. 3** and **6**).

FLUCTUATION SCALING OF ACCELEROMETRIC TIME SERIES

Because scaling behavior is a frequently observed property of biomedical data (**Box 2**), we have recently evaluated accelerometer recordings with high sampling rate in this respect.[93]

Specifically, we have shown that these data also exhibit scaling due to long-term correlated fluctuations. They are characterized by a power-law decay of the spectral power $P(f) \sim f^{-\beta}$ with a spectral exponent $\beta \approx 1.0$ (1/f noise) in a frequency range from 33 Hz to 0.00033 Hz; that is, oscillation periods $T = 1/f$ between 0.03 and 3000 seconds. For this result, however, the respiratory peak (see **Figs. 2** and **3**) had to be excluded. On short time scales between 0.03 and 30 seconds, we observed that β is larger during wake ($\beta \approx 1.4$) and smaller during sleep ($\beta \approx 0.6$): a property

that can be used for distinguishing between these 2 states.

A PERIODOGRAM-BASED SLEEP DETECTION ALGORITHM

We have thus designed a periodogram-based sleep detection (PBSD) algorithm.[93] After calculating the periodogram $P(f)$ for each epoch of 30 seconds, we performed power-law fits (ie, linear fits according to $\log P(f) \approx -\beta \log f + o$ with slope β and offset o), neglecting the peaks from respiration and physiologic tremor (0.2–0.4 Hz and 4–10 Hz, respectively). In addition, the height r of the respiratory peak was calculated by dividing the peak maximum by the average (logarithmic) intensity in the frequency range from 0.1 to 0.4 Hz. Next, we smoothened the time series of slope β, offset o, and respiration strength r values by exponential backward averages, using 2 different exponential decay times for β and o. Finally, a weighted average of the resulting 5 parameters (ie, a linear combination with 5 tuned coefficients), was calculated and compared with a threshold to identify the 30-second epochs as

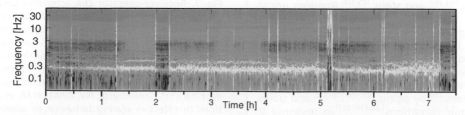

Fig. 5. Time-dependent spectrogram of a nocturnal acceleration recording taken at the hip of a healthy subject, presented the same way as in **Fig. 4**.

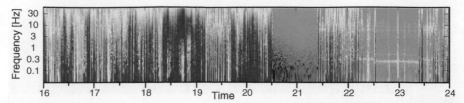

Fig. 6. Time-dependent spectrogram of an acceleration recording taken at the wrist of a healthy subject during the evening (16:00–24:00), presented the same way as in **Fig. 4**.

"sleep" or "wake." The threshold was defined using receiver-operator characteristics curves (**Fig. 7**) during algorithm development. The algorithm was developed using the data of 30 randomly chosen subjects of the GNC pretest recordings[93] and then validated for the remaining 70 data recordings.

Fig. 7 shows the receiver-operator characteristic curves we obtained by varying the value of the threshold for the PBSD algorithm, considering only nighttime data (dotted curve) and full 24-hour data (full curve). The areas under the curve (AUC) are 0.84 and 0.95, respectively. For nighttime acceleration data recorded at the patients' hips, we obtained an AUC of 0.81 with our proposed algorithms (not shown). Slightly better AUC values (0.85 and 0.83 for wrist and hip, respectively) could be obtained if an additional normalization step was introduced (also not shown).

ACCELEROMETRY FOR CHARACTERIZING SLEEP

There are still several limitations of accelerometry-based methods in the deduction of sleep characteristics and the detection of sleep disturbances. These limitations differ between devices,

populations, data analysis algorithms, and sleep characteristics of interest.[43,47–49]

Additionally, the influence of the placement (wrist or trunk) on the validity of the assessment has been debated.[43,46,113] The performance of accelerometers often is evaluated by comparing sleep characteristics derived from concurrent PSG and accelerometry recordings. With the exception of total sleep time (TST), the agreement of accelerometry-based measurements of sleep quality, such as sleep-onset latency, sleep efficiency (SE%), and wake after sleep onset (WASO) with PSG is limited.[43,47]

PRETEST STUDIES FOR THE GERMAN NATIONAL COHORT STUDY

During the preparation of the GNC in 2011, the ActiGraph GT3X+ device and the SOMNOwatch plus device were newly developed 3-axis accelerometers. Because there existed only 1 validation study

---

Box 2
Scaling behavior of biomedical time series

Physiologic systems under neural regulation are often characterized by (fractal) scaling relations.[99] For example, 1/f noise (red noise) or "fractal" $1/f^\beta$ noise (pink noise) is often found in biomedical data, such as the series of time intervals between successive heartbeats,[100–102] breaths,[103,104] and steps.[105,106] Random uncorrelated fluctuations (white noise) correspond to frequency-independent power, that is, $\beta = 0$. It has been shown that the dynamics are modified by different physiologic states, in particular by sleep versus wake[107] and by different sleep stages,[102,104,108] by exercise versus rest,[109] by aging,[103,106,108,110] and under pathologic conditions[106,110–112] in response to changes in the underlying control mechanisms.

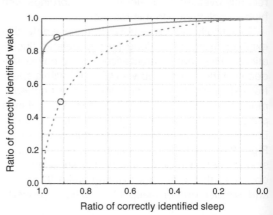

Fig. 7. Receiver-operator characteristics curves based on the accelerometer recordings of 100 subjects, using only nighttime wrist data without normalization (*dotted orange line*) as well as un-normalized daytime and nighttime wrist data (*continuous green*). Points for optimized sleep/wake differentiation thresholds are marked by red circles. (*Data from* Wohlfahrt P, Kantelhardt JW, Zinkhan M, et al. Transitions in effective scaling behavior of accelerometric time series across sleep and wake. Europhys Lett 2013;103(6):68002.)

for the deduction of sleep characteristics with such modern devices,[97] a validation study for both accelerometers was included among the GNC pretest studies.[114,115] We focused on the agreement of sleep characteristics between GT3X+ (sampling rate 80 Hz), SOMNOwatch plus (sampling rate 128 Hz), and PSG instead of comparing classified sleep and wake epochs in terms of sensitivity, specificity, or accuracy. Sleep characteristics were determined with the algorithms[52,97] used in the analysis software provided by the manufacturers. Different placements (wrist, hip) of the devices were also considered. **Fig. 8** shows Bland-Altman plots[116] for the agreement between PSG and SOMNOwatch plus placed at the wrist of 100 individuals (49 men, 51 women, aged 18–75 years).[115]

Specifically, for the evaluation of agreement, we considered mean differences as a measure of systematic error (bias) and 95% limits of agreement as measure of precision. We also evaluated whether the absolute value or the precision of the observed differences depended on the magnitude of the respective measure (see **Fig. 8**).[116] For TST, there is no dependency of the differences between results from PSG and SOMNOwatch plus placed at the wrist on average TST, whereas the numbers of awakenings after sleep onset (NASO) shows higher differences to PSG with increasing average values of NASO. SE and WASO become more precise (SE) or less precise

(WASO) over the range of measurement. Taken together, the agreement with PSG depends on the sleep measure of interest.[115] The decision of whether accelerometry can be used for measuring a particular sleep characteristic for a particular application should take the components of agreement in terms of mean bias, the precision of differences, and the dependency of the measurement errors on the magnitude of the measure into account. For individual diagnostics it might be a problem if the interval between 95% limits of agreement is large, irrespective of a small mean bias for that measure, as can be seen for TST or SE (see **Fig. 8**). However, the assessment of specific sleep measures with accelerometry might be appropriate if population means of sleep measures are of interest, as it is in cohort studies for example.[115]

PLACEMENT OF THE ACCELEROMETER

We would like to note that the placement of accelerometers is crucial for the deduction of sleep measures if algorithms developed and validated for wrist measurements are used.[115] **Fig. 9** shows the same comparisons as **Fig. 8**, but with accelerometers placed at the right side of the hip.[115] Mean bias to PSG is larger, and there is a distinct dependency of the differences on the magnitude of the respective sleep measures. Slater and

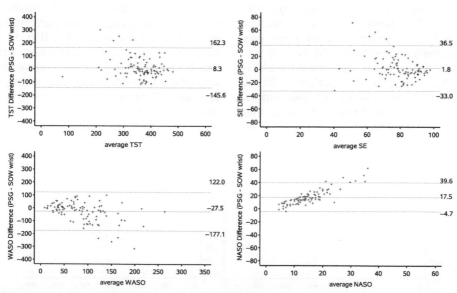

Fig. 8. Difference of sleep characteristics from PSG and SOMNOwatch plus placed at the wrist (SOW wrist) against average of PSG and SOW wrist sleep measurements, with mean difference (*solid line*) and 95% limits of agreement (*broken lines*). Differences are shown in the y-axis and averages in the x-axis. (*Data from* Zinkhan M, Berger K, Hense S, et al. Agreement of different methods for assessing sleep characteristics: a comparison of two actigraphs, wrist and hip placement, and self-report with polysomnography. Sleep Med 2014;15(9):1107–14.)

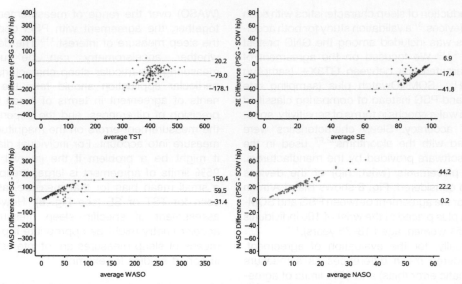

Fig. 9. Difference of sleep characteristics from PSG and SOMNOwatch plus placed at the right hip, presented as in **Fig. 8.** (*Data from* Zinkhan M, Berger K, Hense S, et al. Agreement of different methods for assessing sleep characteristics: a comparison of two actigraphs, wrist and hip placement, and self-report with polysomnography. Sleep Med 2014;15(9):1107–14.)

colleagues[117] recently published similar results for sleep measures based on GT3X+ hip recordings and analyzed with the Sadeh algorithm.[53]

Considering our previous results from spectral analysis,[93] we concluded that the unfavorable differences shown in **Fig. 9** are the result of unsuitable algorithms used for hip recordings instead of an inability for measuring sleep characteristics with accelerometers placed at the hip in general. When studying TST derived from the hip recordings via the PBSD algorithm (**Fig. 10**, right), one can see that the agreement with PSG is comparable with the corresponding agreement for SOMNOwatch plus wrist recordings analyzed with the algorithm by Dick and colleagues[97] (see **Fig. 8**, top left). Taken together, there is evidence that for modern accelerometers, the observed

differences between sleep measures derived by hip-based and wrist-based recordings are the consequence of unsuitable algorithms and not of the inappropriateness of the placement itself.

COMPARISON WITH SELF-REPORTED SLEEP PARAMETERS

We have also compared PSG results with self-reported sleep characteristic parameters, obtaining a Bland-Altman plot for TST (**Fig. 10**, left) quite similar to the plot for the wrist measurements (see **Fig. 8**, top left). This comparison shows that accelerometry is not necessarily superior to self-report, at least as long as there is a low prevalence of sleep disorders. Individuals with insomnia, for example, tend to underestimate their TST

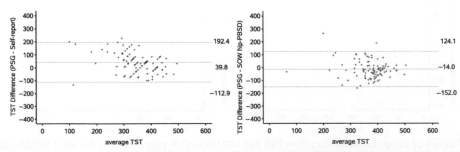

Fig. 10. Difference of PSG-based and self-reported TST (*left*), as well as TST derived by the PBSD algorithm from data recorded by SOMNOwatch plus placed at the hip (SOW hip-PBSD) (*right*) in the same presentation as in **Figs. 8** and **9**. (*From* Wohlfahrt P, Kantelhardt JW, Zinkhan M, et al. Transitions in effective scaling behavior of accelerometric time series across sleep and wake. Europhys Lett 2013;103(6):68002; with permission.)

considerably.[118] If we stratify our results by the Pittsburgh sleep quality index[89] (PSQI, ≤ 5 vs >5) we can see that people with higher PSQI scores underestimate their TST by approximately 60 minutes on average, whereas subjects with PSG scores ≤ 5 underestimate their TST by only 23 minutes on average. The accelerometry-based TST measures are less sensitive to PSQI scores in our population (results not shown), although their accuracy also decreases the more sleep is disturbed.[43,47] Whether this is still true for newly developed algorithms and modern devices has to be evaluated by systematic comparisons to PSG in future studies.

DATA HANDLING IN LARGE COHORT STUDIES

The quantity of high-resolution accelerometry data raises challenges, especially in large-scale multi-center studies, as exemplified by the SOMNO-watch plus recordings of the GNC. The availability of the data in open nonproprietary formats is necessary to enable researchers at different locations and at different points in time to work efficiently with the recorded data. For this reason, the SOMNOwatch plus data of the GNC is exported in European Data Format (220 Mb for each recording). Hence, for a total of 40,000 participants, approximately 8.8 TB of binary data files have to be transferred from the local study centers to the 2 data integration centers and stored there with continuous mutual back-ups.[74]

DATA QUALITY CONTROL IN LARGE COHORT STUDIES

According to the recommendations of Good Epidemiologic Practice (GEP) that claims accompanying quality assurance of all relevant instruments and procedures,[119] we have established a data quality control program for the SOMNOwatch plus recordings for the purpose of sleep evaluation during the initial phase of the GNC study. Specifically, we have identified segments of usable data for all 3 kinds of sensors in each 24-hour recording.

- Accelerometry (g-force in 3 directions recorded at 128 Hz): we identified the total durations and the numbers of episodes when the device was actually worn by a subject; 80% of recording time was chosen as the threshold for high-quality recordings.
- ECG (256 Hz): we identified the total durations and the number of episodes when a signal was recorded with a signal-to-noise ratio sufficient for further analysis; 65% of recording time with a satisfying signal-to-noise ratio

was chosen as threshold for high-quality recordings.
- Nasal pressure (256 Hz, recorded during the night only): we identified the total durations and the numbers of episodes when there was sufficient spectral power in the frequency band associated with respiration (5–30 breaths per minute). At least 10% of the total 24-hour recording time should fulfill these criteria for high-quality recordings.

Most of the initial GNC accelerometer and ECG recordings are satisfying based on these criteria with high-quality recordings per individual exceeding 22 hours on average. Respiratory recordings (nasal pressure) are typically between 6 and 10 hours long, because the sensor is worn during the night only. Although most recordings consist of single (continuous) episodes, there are also some interruptions, most of them regarding the ECG (in nearly half of all recordings). Quality scores were assigned for each high-quality recording (3 points, 1 for each signal), reasonable lights on/off times (1 point), and for a formal check (1 point). The formal check included the duration of the recording, which should be exactly 24 hours. Battery failure turned out to be a particularly prominent cause of shorter durations.

SLEEP ASSESSMENT IN THE GERMAN NATIONAL COHORT COMPARED WITH ALREADY ESTABLISHED COHORTS

Because of the large number of participants and the use of state-of the art technologies, the GNC study will be able to provide a substantial benefit to actual sleep research. Unfortunately, it was not feasible to implement PSG recordings and to perform SOMNOwatch plus recordings for more than 24 hours in the GNC because of the large numbers of participants throughout Germany. Nevertheless, compared with already established cohorts, the GNC will be able to provide one of the largest and most comprehensive sleep assessments that considers subjective information on sleep, as well as objective measures together with concurrent recordings of ECG and respiration.

SUMMARY

Our review article has addressed the properties, challenges, and limitations of accelerometry for the deduction of sleep characteristics in large-scale studies, such as cohort studies. It provides an overview on established cohort studies with objective measurements on sleep, published sleep-wake differentiation algorithms for accelerometer recordings, and discusses unresolved issues for the application of state-of-the-art accelerometers in current large prospective study designs. Specific challenges are exemplified by the application in the GNC study. We have described the newly developed periodogram-based sleep-wake differentiation algorithm that addresses some of these challenges and summarized the results of a GNC pretest study. Additionally, data handling and quality assurance procedures are described for the example of the GNC study.

ACKNOWLEDGMENTS

Some of the presented results were obtained in the context of the pretest studies of the German National Cohort (www.nako.de), see Refs.[67,89] The pretest studies were funded by the Federal Ministry of Education and Research (BMBF, grant 01ER1001A-1) and supported by the Helmholtz Association, as well as by the participating universities and institutes of the Leibniz Association. J.W. Kantelhardt is thankful to the German Research Society (DFG, grant KA 1676/4) and the German-Israeli Foundation (grant I-1298-415.13/2015) for financial support.

REFERENCES

1. Tregear S, Reston J, Schoelles K, et al. Obstructive sleep apnea and risk of motor vehicle crash: systematic review and meta-analysis. J Clin Sleep Med 2009;5(6):573–81.
2. Ohayon MM, Bader G. Prevalence and correlates of insomnia in the Swedish population aged 19-75 years. Sleep Med 2010;11(10):980–6.
3. Ohayon MM, Sagales T. Prevalence of insomnia and sleep characteristics in the general population of Spain. Sleep Med 2010;11(10):1010–8.
4. Philip P, Sagaspe P, Lagarde E, et al. Sleep disorders and accidental risk in a large group of regular registered highway drivers. Sleep Med 2010;11(10):973–9.
5. Cappuccio FP, Taggart FM, Kandala NB, et al. Meta-analysis of short sleep duration and obesity in children and adults. Sleep 2008;31(5):619–26.
6. Vgontzas AN, Liao D, Bixler EO, et al. Insomnia with objective short sleep duration is associated with a high risk for hypertension. Sleep 2009; 32(4):491–7.
7. Wang QJ, Xi B, Liu M, et al. Short sleep duration is associated with hypertension risk among adults: a systematic review and meta-analysis. Hypertens Res 2012;35(10):1012–8.
8. Guo XF, Zheng LQ, Wang J, et al. Epidemiological evidence for the link between sleep duration and high blood pressure: a systematic

9. Moraes W, Poyares D, Zalcman I, et al. Association between body mass index and sleep duration assessed by objective methods in a representative sample of the adult population. Sleep Med 2013; 14(4):312–8.
10. Vgontzas AN, Bixler EO, Chrousos GP. Sleep apnea is a manifestation of the metabolic syndrome. Sleep Med Rev 2005;9(3):211–24.
11. Tuomilehto H, Peltonen M, Partinen M, et al. Sleep duration, lifestyle intervention, and incidence of Type 2 diabetes in impaired glucose tolerance: the Finnish Diabetes Prevention Study. Diabetes Care 2009;32(11):1965–71.
12. Vgontzas AN, Liao D, Pejovic S, et al. Insomnia with objective short sleep duration is associated with type 2 diabetes: a population-based study. Diabetes Care 2009;32(11):1980–5.
13. Xu Q, Song YQ, Hollenbeck A, et al. Day napping and short night sleeping are associated with higher risk of diabetes in older adults. Diabetes Care 2010;33(1):78–83.
14. Cappuccio FP, D'Elia L, Strazzillo P, et al. Quantity and quality of sleep and incidence of type 2 diabetes - a systematic review and meta-analysis. Diabetes Care 2010;33(2):414–20.
15. Chien KL, Chen PC, Hsu HC, et al. Habitual sleep duration and insomnia and the risk of cardiovascular events and all-cause death: report from a community-based cohort. Sleep 2010;33(2): 177–84.
16. Sofi F, Cesari F, Casini A, et al. Insomnia and risk of cardiovascular disease: a meta-analysis. Eur J Prev Cardiol 2014;21(1):57–64.
17. Hublin C, Partinen M, Koskenvuo M, et al. Sleep and mortality: a population-based 22-year follow-up study. Sleep 2007;30(10):1245–53.
18. Gallicchio L, Kalesan B. Sleep duration and mortality: a systematic review and meta-analysis. J Sleep Res 2009;18(2):148–58.
19. Cappuccio FP, D'Elia L, Strazzullo P, et al. Sleep duration and all-cause mortality: a systematic review and meta-analysis of prospective studies. Sleep 2010;33(5):585–92.
20. Vgontzas AN, Liao D, Pejovic S, et al. Insomnia with short sleep duration and mortality: the Penn State cohort. Sleep 2010;33(9):1159–64.
21. Kripke DF, Langer RD, Elliott JA, et al. Mortality related to actigraphic long and short sleep. Sleep Med 2011;12(1):28–33.
22. Guidolin M, Gradisar M. Is shortened sleep duration a risk factor for overweight and obesity during adolescence? A review of the empirical literature. Sleep Med 2012;13(7):779–86.
23. Magee L, Hale L. Longitudinal associations between sleep duration and subsequent weight

gain: a systematic review. Sleep Med Rev 2012; 16(3):231–41.

24. Kurina LM, McClintock MK, Chen J-H, et al. Sleep duration and all-cause mortality: a critical review of measurement and associations. Ann Epidemiol 2013;23(6):361–70.

25. Rechtschaffen A, Kales A. A manual of standardized terminology, techniques, and scoring system for sleep stages of human subjects. Washington, DC: U. S. Public Health Service; 1968.

26. Iber C, Ancoli-Israel A, Chesson AL, et al. The AASM manual for the scoring of sleep and associated events: rules, terminology and technical specifications. 1st edition. Westchester (IL): American Academy of Sleep Medicine; 2007.

27. Berry RB, Brooks R, Gamaldo CE, et al. The AASM manual for the scoring of sleep and associated events. rules, terminology and technical specifications, version 2.0. Darien (IL): American Academy of Sleep Medicine; 2012.

28. Berry RB, Brooks R, Gamaldo CE, et al. The AASM manual for the scoring of sleep and associated events. rules, terminology and technical specifications, version 2.2. Darien (IL): American Academy of Sleep Medicine; 2015.

29. Ferrie JE, Kumari M, Salo P, et al. Sleep epidemiology—a rapidly growing field. Int J Epidemiol 2011;40(6):1431–7.

30. Agnew HW, Webb WB, Williams RL. The first night effect: an EEG study of sleep. Psychophysiology 1966;2(3):263–6.

31. Curcio G, Ferrara M, Piergianni A, et al. Paradoxes of the first-night effect: a quantitative analysis of antero-posterior EEG topography. Clin Neurophysiol 2004;115(5):1178–88.

32. Goel N, Kim H, Lao RP. Gender differences in polysomnographic sleep in young healthy sleepers. Chronobiol Int 2005;22(5):905–15.

33. Szklo-Coxe M, Young T, Peppard PE, et al. Prospective associations of insomnia markers and symptoms with depression. Am J Epidemiol 2010; 171(6):709–20.

34. Edinger JD, Fins AI, Sullivan RJ, et al. Sleep in the laboratory and sleep at home: comparisons of older insomniacs and normal sleepers. Sleep 1997;20(12):1119–26.

35. Edinger JD, Glenn DM, Bastian LA, et al. Sleep in the laboratory and sleep at home II: comparisons of middle-aged insomnia sufferers and normal sleepers. Sleep 2001;24(7):761–70.

36. Silva GE, Goodwin JL, Sherrill DL, et al. Relationship between reported and measured sleep times: the sleep heart health study (SHHS). J Clin Sleep Med 2007;3(6):622–30.

37. Bruyneel M, Sanida C, Art G, et al. Sleep efficiency during sleep studies: results of a prospective study

comparing home-based and in-hospital polysomnography. J Sleep Res 2011;20(1):201–6.

38. Kupfer DJ, Weiss BL, Foster FG, et al. Psychomotor activity in affective states. Arch Gen Psychiatry 1974;30(6):765–8.

39. McPartland RJ, Kupfer DJ, Foster FG. Movement-activated recording monitor: 3rd-generation motor-activity monitoring-system. Behav Res Meth Instr 1976;8(4):357–60.

40. Colburn TR, Smith BM, Guarini JJ, et al. Ambulatory activity monitor with solid-state memory. ISA Trans 1976;15(2):149–54.

41. Koenig SM, Mack D, Alwan M. Sleep and sleep assessment technologies. In: Alwan M, Felder RA, editors. Eldercare technology for clinical practitioners. New York: Humana Press; 2008. p. 77–120.

42. Tryon WW. Equipment used for measuring activity. Activity measurement in psychology and medicine. New York: Plenum Press; 1991. p. 23–55.

43. Ancoli-Israel S, Cole R, Alessi C, et al. The role of actigraphy in the study of sleep and circadian rhythms. Sleep 2003;26(3):342–92.

44. McCall C, McCall WV. Objective vs. subjective measurements of sleep in depressed insomniacs: first night effect or reverse first night effect? J Clin Sleep Med 2012;8(1):59–65.

45. Godfrey A, Conway R, Meagher D, et al. Direct measurement of human movement by accelerometry. Med Eng Phys 2008;30(10):1364–86.

46. Sadeh A, Hauri PJ, Kripke DF, et al. The role of actigraphy in the evaluation of sleep disorders. Sleep 1995;18(4):288–302.

47. Sadeh A, Acebo C. The role of actigraphy in sleep medicine. Sleep Med Rev 2002;6(2):113–24.

48. Lichstein KL, Stone KC, Donaldson J, et al. Actigraphy validation with insomnia. Sleep 2006;29(2): 232–9.

49. van de Water ATM, Holmes A, Hurley DA. Objective measurements of sleep for non-laboratory settings as alternatives to polysomnography: a systematic review. J Sleep Res 2011;20(1):183–200.

50. Kushida CA, Littner MR, Morgenthaler T, et al. Practice parameters for the indications for polysomnography and related procedures: an update for 2005. Sleep 2005;28(4):499–521.

51. Morgenthaler T, Alessi C, Friedman L, et al. Practice parameters for the use of actigraphy in the assessment of sleep and sleep disorders: an update for 2007. Sleep 2007;30(4):519–29.

52. Cole RJ, Kripke DF, Gruen W, et al. Automatic sleep/wake identification from wrist activity. Sleep 1992;15(5):461–9.

53. Sadeh A, Sharkey KM, Carskadon MA. Activity-based sleep-wake identification: an empirical-test of methodological issues. Sleep 1994;17(3):201–7.

54. Nakazaki K, Kitamura S, Motomura Y, et al. Validity of an algorithm for determining sleep/wake states

using a new actigraph. J Physiol Anthropol 2014; 33:31.

55. Galland B, Kennedy G, Mitchell E, et al. Activity-based accelerometry for identification of infant sleep-wake states: trial of a new algorithm and investigation of performance and accuracy. J Sleep Res 2012;21:218–9.

56. Enomoto M, Endo T, Suenaga K, et al. Newly developed waist actigraphy and its sleep/wake scoring algorithm. Sleep Biol Rhythms 2009;7(1):17–22.

57. Kripke DF, Hahn EK, Grizas AP, et al. Wrist actigraphic scoring for sleep laboratory patients: algorithm development. J Sleep Res 2010;19(4):612–9.

58. Hedner J, Pillar G, Pittman SD, et al. A novel adaptive wrist actigraphy algorithm for sleep-wake assessment in sleep apnea patients. Sleep 2004; 27(8):1560–6.

59. Bixler EO, Kales A, Soldatos CR, et al. Prevalence of sleep disorders in the Los-Angeles metropolitan area. Am J Psychiatry 1979;136(10):1257–62.

60. Riboli E, Kaaks R. The EPIC project: rationale and study design. Int J Epidemiol 1997;26:S6–14.

61. National Health and Nutrition Examination Survey (NHANES) study group. National Health and Nutrition Examination Survey Questionnaire (or Examination Protocol, or Laboratory Protocol). MD: U.S. Department of Health and Human Services, Centers for Disease Control and Prevention; 2016. Available at: http://www.cdc.gov/nchs/data/nhanes/survey_content_99_16.pdf. Accessed July 28, 2016.

62. Allen N, Sudlow C, Downey P, et al. UK Biobank: current status and what it means for epidemiology. Health Policy Techn 2012;1(3):123–6.

63. Scholtens S, Smidt N, Swertz MA, et al. Cohort profile: lifelines, a three-generation cohort study and biobank. Int J Epidemiol 2015;44(4):1172–80.

64. LifeGene study group. Description of the LifeGene Resource. Version 2.3. 2016. Available at: https://www.lifegene.se/PageFiles/591/LifeGene%20resource%2020160226.pdf. Accessed August 1, 2016.

65. Young T, Palta M, Dempsey J, et al. The occurrence of sleep-disordered breathing among middle-aged adults. N Engl J Med 1993;328(17): 1230–5.

66. Bearpark H, Elliott L, Grunstein R, et al. Snoring and sleep apnea. A population study in Australian men. Am J Respir Crit Care Med 1995;151(5): 1459–65.

67. Quan SF, Howard BV, Iber C, et al. The sleep heart health study: design, rationale, and methods. Sleep 1997;20(12):1077–85.

68. Bixler EO, Vgontzas AN, Ten Have T, et al. Effects of age on sleep apnea in men I. Prevalence and severity. Am J Respir Crit Care Med 1998;157(1): 144–8.

69. Blackwell T, Redline S, Ancoli-Israel S, et al. Comparison of sleep parameters from actigraphy and polysomnography in older women: the SOF study. Sleep 2008;31(2):283–91.

70. Blackwell T, Ancoli-Israel S, Redline S, et al, Osteoporotic Fractures in Men (MrOS) Study Group. Factors that may influence the classification of sleep-wake by wrist actigraphy: the MrOS sleep study. J Clin Sleep Med 2011;7(4):357–67.

71. Schmermund A, Mohlenkamp S, Stang A, et al. Assessment of clinically silent atherosclerotic disease and established and novel risk factors for predicting myocardial infarction and cardiac death in healthy middle-aged subjects: rationale and design of the Heinz Nixdorf RECALL Study. Am Heart J 2002;144(2):212–8.

72. Volzke H, Alte D, Schmidt CO, et al. Cohort profile: the study of health in Pomerania. Int J Epidemiol 2011;40(2):294–307.

73. Loeffler M, Engel C, Ahnert P, et al. The LIFE-Adult-Study: objectives and design of a population-based cohort study with 10,000 deeply phenotyped adults in Germany. BMC Public Health 2015;15:691.

74. Consortium GNCG. The German National Cohort: aims, study design and organization. Eur J Epidemiol 2014;29(5):371–82.

75. Young T. Rationale, design and findings from the Wisconsin Sleep Cohort Study: toward understanding the total societal burden of sleep disordered breathing. Sleep Med Clin 2009;4(1):37–46.

76. Marshall NS, Wong KK, Liu PY, et al. Sleep apnea as an independent risk factor for all-cause mortality: the Busselton Health Study. Sleep 2008;31(8):1079.

77. Bixler EO, Vgontzas AN, Lin HM, et al. Prevalence of sleep-disordered breathing in women: effects of gender. Am J Respir Crit Care Med 2001;163(3): 608–13.

78. Redline S, Sanders MH, Lind BK, et al. Methods for obtaining and analyzing unattended polysomnography data for a multicenter study. Sleep Heart Health Research Group. Sleep 1998;21(7): 759–67.

79. Jean-Louis G, Kripke DF, Mason WJ, et al. Sleep estimation from wrist movement quantified by different actigraphic modalities. J Neurosci Methods 2001;105(2):185–91.

80. Blank JB, Cawthon PM, Carrion-Petersen ML, et al. Overview of recruitment for the osteoporotic fractures in men study (MrOS). Contemp Clin Trials 2005;26(5):557–68.

81. Weinreich G, Wessendorf TE, Erdmann T, et al. Association of obstructive sleep apnoea with subclinical coronary atherosclerosis. Atherosclerosis 2013;231(2):191–7.

82. Heinzer R, Vat S, Marques-Vidal P, et al. Prevalence of sleep-disordered breathing in the general population: the HypnoLaus study. Lancet Respir Med 2015;3(4):310–8.

83. UK Biobank Study Group. Category 2 enhanced phenotyping at baseline assessment visit in last 100–150,000 participants. Addendum to main study protocol. 2009. Available at: http://www.ukbiobank.ac.uk/wp-content/uploads/2011/06/Protocol_addendum_2.pdf. Accessed July 27, 2016.

84. UK Biobank Study Group. Physical activity monitor (accelerometer). Version 1.0. 2016. Available at: http://biobank.ctsu.ox.ac.uk/crystal/docs/Physical ActivityMonitor.pdf. Accessed July 27, 2016.

85. Spada J, Scholz M, Kirsten H, et al. Genome-wide association analysis of actigraphic sleep phenotypes in the LIFE Adult Study. J Sleep Res 2016. [Epub ahead of print].

86. Wichmann HE, Horlein A, Ahrens W, et al. The biobank of the German National Cohort as a resource for epidemiologic research. Bundesgesundheitsblatt Gesundheitsforschung Gesundheitsschutz 2016;59(3):351–60 [in German].

87. Bamberg F, Kauczor HU, Weckbach S, et al. Whole-body MR imaging in the German National Cohort: rationale, design, and technical background. Radiology 2015;277(1):206–20.

88. Stallmann C, Ahrens W, Kaaks R, et al. Individual linkage of primary data with secondary and registry data within large cohort studies—capabilities and procedural proposals. Gesundheitswesen 2015; 77(2):e37–42 [in German].

89. Buysse DJ, Reynolds CF 3rd, Monk TH, et al. The Pittsburgh Sleep Quality Index: a new instrument for psychiatric practice and research. Psychiatry Res 1989;28(2):193–213.

90. Netzer NC, Stoohs RA, Netzer CM, et al. Using the Berlin Questionnaire to identify patients at risk for the sleep apnea syndrome. Ann Intern Med 1999; 131(7):485–91.

91. Griefahn B, Künemund C, Bröde P, et al. Zur Validität der deutschen Übersetzung des Morningness-Eveningness-Questionnaires von Horne und Östberg. Somnologie 2001;5(2):71–80.

92. Horne JA, Ostberg O. A self-assessment questionnaire to determine morningness-eveningness in human circadian rhythms. Int J Chronobiol 1976; 4(2):97–110.

93. Wohlfahrt P, Kantelhardt JW, Zinkhan M, et al. Transitions in effective scaling behavior of accelerometric time series across sleep and wake. Europhys Lett 2013;103(6):68002.

94. de Souza L, Benedito-Silva AA, Pires ML, et al. Further validation of actigraphy for sleep studies. Sleep 2003;26(1):81–5.

95. Gorny S, Allen R, Krausman D, et al. Parametric analyses of factors affecting accuracy for detection of wake epochs after sleep onset based on wrist activity data. Sleep Res 1996;25:490.

96. Gorny S, Allen R, Krausmann D, et al. A parametric and sleep hysteresis approach to assessing sleep and wake from wrist activity meter with enhanced frequency range. Sleep Res 1997;26:662.

97. Dick R, Penzel T, Fietze I, et al. AASM standards of practice compliant validation of actigraphic sleep analysis from SOMNOwatch versus polysomnographic sleep diagnostics shows high conformity also among subjects with sleep disordered breathing. Physiol Meas 2010;31(12):1623–33.

98. Jean-Louis G, Kripke DF, Cole RJ, et al. Sleep detection with an accelerometer actigraph: comparisons with polysomnography. Physiol Behav 2001;72(1–2):21–8.

99. Bassingthwaighte JB, Liebovitch LS, West BJ. Fractal physiology. New York: Oxford University Press; 1994.

100. Kobayashi M, Musha T. 1/f fluctuation of heartbeat period. IEEE Trans Biomed Eng 1982;29(6):456–7.

101. Peng CK, Mietus J, Hausdorff JM, et al. Long-range anticorrelations and non-Gaussian behavior of the heartbeat. Phys Rev Lett 1993; 70(9):1343–6.

102. Bunde A, Havlin S, Kantelhardt JW, et al. Correlated and uncorrelated regions in heart-rate fluctuations during sleep. Phys Rev Lett 2000;85(17): 3736–9.

103. Peng C-K, Mietus JE, Liu Y, et al. Quantifying fractal dynamics of human respiration: age and gender effects. Ann Biomed Eng 2002;30(5): 683–92.

104. Kantelhardt JW, Penzel T, Rostig S, et al. Breathing during REM and non-REM sleep: correlated versus uncorrelated behaviour. Phys Stat Mech Appl 2003;319:447–57.

105. Hausdorff JM, Peng C, Ladin Z, et al. Is walking a random walk? Evidence for long-range correlations in stride interval of human gait. J Appl Physiol 1995;78(1):349–58.

106. Hausdorff JM, Mitchell SL, Firtion R, et al. Altered fractal dynamics of gait: reduced stride-interval correlations with aging and Huntington's disease. J Appl Physiol 1997;82(1):262–9.

107. Ivanov PC, Bunde A, Amaral LAN, et al. Sleep-wake differences in scaling behavior of the human heartbeat: analysis of terrestrial and long-term space flight data. Europhys Lett 1999; 48(5):594–600.

108. Schumann AY, Bartsch RP, Penzel T, et al. Aging effects on cardiac and respiratory dynamics in healthy subjects across sleep stages. Sleep 2010;33(7):943–55.

109. Karasik R, Sapir N, Ashkenazy Y, et al. Correlation differences in heartbeat fluctuations during rest and exercise. Phys Rev E 2002;66(6):062902.

110. Goldberger AL, Amaral LA, Hausdorff JM, et al. Fractal dynamics in physiology: alterations with disease and aging. Proc Natl Acad Sci U S A 2002;99(Suppl 1):2466–72.

111. Peng CK, Havlin S, Stanley HE, et al. Quantification of scaling exponents and crossover phenomena in nonstationary heartbeat time-series. Chaos 1995; 5(1):82–7.

112. Seely AJE, Macklem PT. Complex systems and the technology of variability analysis. Crit Care 2004; 8(6):R367–84.

113. Hjorth MF, Chaput J-P, Damsgaard CT, et al. Measure of sleep and physical activity by a single accelerometer: can a waist-worn Actigraph adequately measure sleep in children? Sleep Biol Rhythms 2012;10(4):328–35.

114. Ahrens W, Greiser H, Linseisen J, et al. The design of a nationwide cohort study in Germany: the pretest studies of the German National Cohort (GNC). Bundesgesundheitsblatt Gesundheitsforschung Gesundheitsschutz 2014;57(11):1246–54 [in German].

115. Zinkhan M, Berger K, Hense S, et al. Agreement of different methods for assessing sleep characteristics: a comparison of two actigraphs, wrist and hip placement, and self-report with polysomnography. Sleep Med 2014;15(9):1107–14.

116. Bland JM, Altman DG. Statistical methods for assessing agreement between two methods of clinical measurement. Lancet 1986;1(8476):307–10.

117. Slater JA, Botsis T, Walsh J, et al. Assessing sleep using hip and wrist actigraphy. Sleep Biol Rhythms 2015;13(2):172–80.

118. Manconi M, Ferri R, Sagrada C, et al. Measuring the error in sleep estimation in normal subjects and in patients with insomnia. J Sleep Res 2010;19(3):478–86.

119. Hoffmann W, Latza U, Terschüren C. Guidelines and recommendations for ensuring Good Epidemiological Practice (GEP)—revised version after evaluation. Gesundheitswesen 2005;67(3):217 [in German].

Model-Derived Markers of Autonomic Cardiovascular Dysfunction in Sleep-Disordered Breathing

Michael C.K. Khoo, PhD*, Patjanaporn Chalacheva, PhD

KEYWORDS

- Heart rate variability • Cardiorespiratory control • Minimal model • Sleep apnea
- Peripheral vascular resistance

KEY POINTS

- A large body of evidence suggests that abnormal autonomic control is an important causal link between sleep-disordered breathing (SDB) and cardiovascular disease.
- Heart rate variability and peripheral arterial tonometry have been used to detect and assess autonomic changes in SDB, but the mechanistic information derived from these techniques is limited by the univariate nature of the underlying analyses.
- An alternative approach is to use multivariate dynamic models that enable the causal dependencies among respiration, blood pressure, heart rate variability, and peripheral vascular resistance to be quantified, and from which compact descriptors ("biophysical markers") are derived.
- The model-derived markers representing respiratory-cardiac coupling, baroreflex control of heart rate, and blood pressure modulation of peripheral vascular resistance are significantly altered in patients with SDB during wakefulness and sleep.

INTRODUCTION AND BACKGROUND

Several large epidemiologic studies have suggested that sleep-disordered breathing (SDB), which occurs most commonly in the form of obstructive sleep apnea (OSA), constitutes an independent risk factor for the development of a wide range of cardiovascular diseases.[1,2] For instance, the Wisconsin Sleep Cohort Study, with more than 700 subjects, demonstrated that the adjusted odds ratio of incident systemic hypertension in SDB subjects with respiratory disturbance index greater than 15 was almost 3 times higher relative to subjects without SDB.[3] In the Sleep Heart Health Study cohort of 6132 subjects, SDB was found to be strongly correlated with coronary heart disease, heart failure, and stroke.[4] Nieto and colleagues[5] found the odds ratio of hypertension to increase with severity of SDB. Studies using animal models have been useful in suggesting causal links between the key acute effects of SDB—intermittent hypoxia and sleep disruption—and its chronic cardiovascular sequelae.[6] Brooks and colleagues[7] were able to produce nocturnal and daytime hypertension by exposing a dog model to sleep-triggered periodic airway obstructions for several weeks. On the other hand, sustained exposure to periodic acoustically induced arousals without accompanying airway obstruction in these animals produced only nocturnal hypertension with no carryover effect in the daytime. In a rat model, Fletcher and colleagues[8,9] found that sustained hypertension developed after a few weeks

Biomedical Engineering Department, University of Southern California, 1042 Downey Way, Los Angeles, CA 90089, USA
* Corresponding author.
E-mail address: khoo@usc.edu

Sleep Med Clin 11 (2016) 489–501
http://dx.doi.org/10.1016/j.jsmc.2016.07.003
1556-407X/16/© 2016 Elsevier Inc. All rights reserved.

of exposure to intermittent hypoxia without any accompanying upper airway obstruction.

There are several mechanisms through which intermittent hypoxia, produced by SDB, can lead to hypertension and other forms of cardiovascular disease, but abnormal autonomic control appears to play a major role.[10,11] Studies using peroneal microneurography or testing of plasma catecholamines have shown that sympathetic tone is abnormally high in subjects with SDB in both sleep and wakefulness.[12,13] Narkiewicz and colleagues[14] compared obese adult subjects with and without SDB and showed that obesity alone, in the absence of SDB, was not accompanied by increased muscle sympathetic nerve activity. Treatment with continuous positive airway pressure (CPAP) partially reverses these effects.[15–18]

To determine whether the abnormal autonomic control is causally related to the exposure to intermittent hypoxia, several prospective studies in normal humans have been carried out. Xie and colleagues[19] found that exposing healthy young subjects to intermittent asphyxia over a period of 20 minutes led to sympathetic activation that continued even after the stimulus was removed. In another study, prolonged sympathetic activation was produced after 20 minutes of exposure to intermittent hypoxic apnea.[20] The results were similar regardless of whether these exposures occurred against a background of hypercapnia or isocapnia, confirming that the primary mediator for the increase in sympathetic activity was the intermittent hypoxia. Healthy young subjects exposed to repetitive hypoxic apneas displayed small postrecovery elevations in mean arterial blood pressure, along with a more sustained and substantial increase in muscle sympathetic nerve activity.[21,22] Baroreflex impairment resulting from SDB could also be involved in the development of altered vasoconstrictor function and systemic hypertension.[23] Narkiewicz and colleagues[24] found abnormal baroreflex sympathetic modulation in subjects with SDB. The authors' studies have shown reduced baroreflex control of heart rate in patients with SDB,[25] which was partially restored following long-term CPAP therapy.[26]

"SIGNALS" VERSUS "SYSTEMS" ANALYSIS

The association between SDB and autonomic dysfunction suggests that the monitoring of the relevant autonomic variables may constitute a useful means of tracking the development of the disorder over time in individual subjects. Peroneal microneurography provides the most direct measurement of muscle sympathetic nerve activity, but the method is impractical in terms of clinical utility because it requires considerable technical expertise and is highly susceptible to artifactual noise introduced by limb movements.[27] Plasma or urinary catecholamine concentrations provide an integrated measure of sympathetic outflow over a period of many hours, and as such, are limited in sensitivity and temporal resolution.[28] Cardiovascular stress tests are relatively easy to administer clinically, but they have been shown to be rather insensitive and require subject cooperation, which is not possible during sleep.[29]

Assessment of autonomic nervous system activity using heart rate variability (HRV) has attained widespread popularity due to the ease, noninvasiveness, and nonintrusiveness of obtaining the measurements on a continuous basis over significant lengths of time, including during sleep, because subject cooperation is not necessary. The present consensus is that only parasympathetic (vagal) activity accounts for the contribution to the high-frequency (HF, 0.15–0.4 Hz) component of HRV.[30] On the other hand, the low-frequency (LF, 0.04–0.15 Hz) component of HRV can be due to both vagal and sympathetic activities.[31] The ratio between LF and HF spectral powers has been used by researchers broadly as an index of "sympathovagal balance."[32] The premise that HRV can provide useful indices of cardiac autonomic control may be traced back to Katona and Jih,[33] who demonstrated, in an anesthetized dog preparation, a linear relationship between vagal firing rate and RR interval (RRI), the inverse of beat-to-beat heart rate. Their finding was obtained under conditions in which respiration was relatively well controlled. Subsequent studies extended this notion to humans, and pharmacologic interventions were used to alter the relative importance of sympathetic versus vagal modulation of heart rate. In these studies, respiration was either controlled or kept relatively uniform while vagal activity was altered. However, the natural variability in respiration, particularly during changes in sleep-wake state, can seriously confound the presumed simple relationship between RRI and vagal traffic.[34,35] Moreover, changes in ventilation and ventilatory pattern can alter autonomic input to the heart via chemoreceptor feedback. As well, changes in breathing alter vagal feedback from the lungs, and this has been shown to influence sympathetic activity.

Another major drawback of using HRV alone to assess autonomic function is that one can only derive from this information the net effect of all the factors that contribute to heart rate control, thus providing little insight into the underlying physiologic mechanisms. One way of overcoming the limitations inherent in univariate signal analysis is to measure other related signals in parallel and to use multivariate analysis to determine how each signal may be related to the others. A prime example is the "alpha index," which represents the gain of the transfer function relating blood pressure variability (or more specifically, changes in systolic blood pressure [SBP]) to changes in RRI. Thus, instead of deriving information from HRV or blood pressure variability as individual signals, this "systems" approach allows one to extract the dynamic properties of the "black box" that relates fluctuations in RRI to fluctuations in blood pressure. However, although the alpha index is frequently used as a measure of baroreflex sensitivity,[36] this presumption ignores the fact that RRI and blood pressure are physiologically coupled to one another in a closed-loop system: changes in blood pressure produce changes in RRI via the baroreflexes, but changes in RRI can also lead to changes in blood pressure through variations in cardiac output via Starling's law and the Windkessel effect.[37] Moreover, because the alpha index represents a one-input one-output system (blood pressure to RRI), it also does not include the effects of other inputs, such as respiration. Thus, in order to take into account multiple inputs and feedback in a given system, it is necessary to formulate a model that contains explicit functional pathways that reflect physiologic dependencies among the various variables (eg, RRI, blood pressure, respiration). Each component in this model can have multiple inputs, but the dynamics between each input and the output must be "causal," that is, changes in the output at the present time can only be ascribed to changes in one or more of the inputs that occurred in the past. Moreover, such a model would be labeled a "minimal model," if it is able to account for most of the dynamic features of a set of physiologic responses and yet be simple enough that all its characteristic parameters can be estimated from measurements obtained in individual subjects.

MODEL-DERIVED MARKERS OF HEART RATE VARIABILITY

Based on knowledge of the underlying physiology, RRI, respiration, and SBP are assumed to be interrelated through the closed-loop control scheme illustrated in **Fig. 1**. Respiration influences RRI directly through autonomic respiratory-cardiac coupling (RCC). The latter includes the mechanisms responsible for central respiratory entrainment of the cardiovagal motor neurons in the medulla as well as vagal feedback from the pulmonary stretch receptors.[38] Respiration also affects RRI indirectly through changes in intrathoracic pressure, which are translated into changes in blood pressure; the latter subsequently stimulate the baroreceptors, leading to fluctuations in RRI. The totality of these respiratory influences on HRV constitutes respiratory sinus arrhythmia. The "closed-loop" nature of the control scheme derives from the fact that changes in RRI, along with changes in stroke volume (not measured), lead to fluctuations in cardiac output that, in turn, produce fluctuations in SBP. Apart from intrathoracic pressure changes and changes in cardiac output, fluctuations in SBP can also arise from other sources of spontaneous variability, such as sympathetically driven variations in peripheral vascular resistance. The part of this closed-loop circulatory control model that accounts for HRV is represented as the area circumscribed by the box (broken lines) displayed in **Fig. 1**. Fluctuations in RRI (ΔRRI) are decomposed into 3 components: the first arising from direct "RCC", the second from

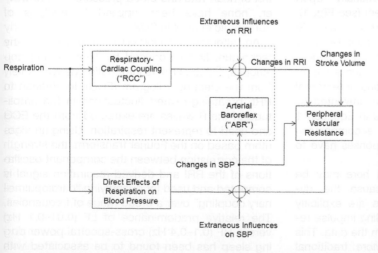

Fig. 1. Schematic block diagram of the closed-loop minimal model of heart rate and blood pressure variability. Fluctuations in RRI result from RCC and a component mediated through the ABR. Other factors are represented as "extraneous influences on RRI." These components account for the "forward" part of the model that generates HRV (rectangular block with broken lines). The "other half" of the closed-loop model consists of the components responsible for generating blood pressure variability: fluctuations in cardiac output (from heart rate and stroke volume changes), fluctuations in peripheral vascular resistance, and respiration.

stimulation of the baroreflexes ("ABR") by variations in blood pressure (ΔSBP), and the third from spontaneous variations not related to respiration (ΔV) or the baroreflexes ("extraneous influences on RRI").

Thus, the HRV part of the model can be characterized mathematically as

$$\Delta RRI(t) = \sum_{\tau = 0}^{P} h_{RCC}(\tau)\Delta V(t - \tau)$$
$$+ \sum_{\tau = 0}^{P} h_{ABR}(\tau)\Delta SBP(t - \tau) + \varepsilon_{RRI}(t)$$

(1)

where $\varepsilon_{RRI}(t)$ represents the totality of contributions to $\Delta RRI(t)$ not accounted for by the postulated mechanisms, including random noise. The dynamics of the RCC and ABR mechanisms are represented by their corresponding impulse responses $h_{RCC}(\tau)$ and $h_{ABR}(\tau)$, which may also include latencies embedded in the responses. In linear systems theory, the impulse response provides a complete characterization of the dynamic properties of the system in question, because the response of this system to any arbitrary input can be predicted by mathematically convolving the input with the impulse response.[39] $h_{ABR}(\tau)$, for instance, quantifies the time course of the change in RRI resulting from an abrupt increase in SBP of 1 mm Hg, whereas $h_{RCC}(\tau)$ quantifies the time course of the fluctuation in RRI associated with a very rapid inspiration and expiration of 1 L of air. It is important to note that, because respiration, RRI, and SBP are measured, it is possible to estimate both model impulse responses from the data. The impulse responses are assumed to be of finite duration (p sampling intervals). An important feature of this model is that its causal structure allows one to computationally "open the loop" of the closed-loop system (see **Fig. 1**), thereby separating the feedforward (ie, how RRI depends on SBP) from the feedback (ie, how SBP depends on RRI) components. Frequency-domain techniques, using spectra derived from RRI and SBP, do not permit this kind of temporal delineation, but this problem is circumvented by solving for the impulse responses in Equation 1 in the time domain, with the accompanying constraint that these impulse responses have to be causal.[39]

The minimal model presented here may be considered "kernel-based," because the dynamics of its major components are explicitly characterized by their corresponding impulse responses, which are estimated from the data. This technique contrasts with the more traditional

approach in which the dynamics are more compactly described using differential equations with unknown coefficients that represent the parameters to be estimated. In order to reduce the level of parametrization and thus increase estimation accuracy, the impulse response of each model component is constructed from the sum of weighted basis functions:

$$h_{ABR}(\tau) = \sum_{j=0}^{q-1} c_j^{ABR} B_j(\tau)$$

(2)

where the $B_j(\tau)$ represents the j-th order orthonormal basis function, and c_j^{ABR} are the corresponding unknown weights that are assigned to $B_j(\tau)$ in the ABR impulse response, with q being the total number of basis functions used. $B_j(\tau)$ may take the form of the Laguerre[40] or Meixner[41] set of functions. The important practical advantage of this computational feature is that these basis functions are predetined, and thus, the only unknown parameters that need to be estimated are the weights c_j^{ABR}. This simplification can produce a substantial reduction in complexity of the estimation process, from p to q, where $p \gg q$, thereby allowing greater statistical reliability to be achieved in the parameter estimates. The reduction in number of parameters estimated is generally on the order of 10-fold. Details of this kernel expansion method are given in Belozeroff and colleagues[25] for Laguerre basis functions and Chaicharn and colleagues[42] for Meixner basis functions. This "minimal model" approach allows one to obtain a comprehensive assessment of the primary mechanisms that contribute to HRV, using data measured from a single test procedure lasting between 5 and 10 minutes. Similar approaches, with individual differences in model structure, have been used to investigate the control of heart rate and blood pressure[43–45]; however, none have been applied to analysis of autonomic control in SDB.

An alternative "minimalist" approach is the technique, first introduced by Thomas and colleagues,[46] that extracts information derived solely from the electrocardiogram (ECG). In addition to RRI, breathing-related fluctuations in the amplitude of the R waves are extracted from the ECG and used to represent respiration. Using an algorithm based on the Fourier transform, the strength of the correlation between the component oscillations of the RRI and derived respiration signal is computed and used for quantifying "cardiopulmonary coupling" over a broad range of frequencies. The relative predominance of LF (0.01–0.1 Hz) versus HF (0.1–0.4 Hz) cross-spectral power during sleep has been found to be associated with higher prevalence of hypertension and stroke in patients with SDB.[47] This approach quantifies cardiorespiratory coupling in the frequency domain, whereas the authors' approach uses a parametric model that is estimated in the time domain. One drawback of the cardiopulmonary coupling technique is that it does not explicitly take into account the component of RRI variability that is mediated by the baroreflexes.

Derivation of Model-Based "Markers"

In the minimal model of HRV, following the estimation of each model impulse response, its corresponding frequency-domain characteristics (ie, its transfer function) can be computed by applying the fast Fourier transform to the impulse response. Compact descriptors of the estimated impulse response or transfer function are subsequently extracted, allowing for statistical comparison across individual or group datasets. These descriptors constitute the model-derived markers associated with the dynamic model that best represents autonomic control under a certain set of conditions (eg, disease vs no disease, predominantly sympathetic vs predominantly vagal, and so forth). For instance, the difference between peak overshoot and peak undershoot is used to represent impulse response magnitude. Another descriptor is the characteristic time, which provides a quantification of how sluggish the impulse response is; thus, a short characteristic time would reflect a highly rapid response to the abrupt stimulus. A third descriptor is the "dynamic gain," which is derived by transforming the impulse response into the equivalent transfer function in the frequency domain and deducing the average gain in the range of frequencies that span the LF and HF regions. In the authors' previous work, these descriptors generally consisted of the following: (1) the LF gain, the average transfer function magnitude between 0.04 and 0.15 Hz; (2) the HF gain, the average transfer function magnitude between 0.15 and 0.4 Hz; and (3) the overall dynamic gain, the average transfer function magnitude between 0.04 and 0.4 Hz.

Application of Heart Rate Variability Minimal Model to Sleep-Disordered Breathing: Summary of Results

The studies that the authors have conducted with the minimal model suggest that it provides a clearer and more mechanistic delineation of sympathetic versus vagal influences on heart rate control than univariate analyses of HRV. For example, an increase in LF and/or HF gains of the RCC component would be consistent with an increase

in vagal tone. Reduced ABR gain would be consistent with elevated sympathetic tone and/or a decrease in vagal tone. This inference is compatible with other studies that have demonstrated impaired baroreflex function in essential hypertension,[48] in congestive heart failure,[49] and following myocardial infarction,[50] all conditions in which sympathetic tone is abnormally elevated. Whether baroreflex dysfunction leads to abnormally high sympathetic tone or chronic exposure to elevated sympathetic drive leads to depressed baroreflex gain remains unresolved at the present time; nevertheless, there is ample evidence that suggests a strong association between depressed baroreflex gain and high sympathetic tone.[49] The studies the authors have performed on human subjects with SDB under a variety of conditions point to a reduction in vagal tone and elevation of sympathetic drive, as detailed below:

a. Patients with moderate-to-severe OSA (apnea-hypopnea index >20) and normal controls were studied during wakefulness under spontaneous breathing conditions in both supine and standing postures. ABR and RCC gains were lower in the SDB subjects relative to controls, and both gains decreased significantly from supine to standing postures.[25] The finding of reduction in gains with orthostatic stress is consistent with the well-known observation that changing posture from supine to standing leads to greater sympathetic dominance and decreased vagal modulation of the heart.

b. Patients with moderate to severe OSA were evaluated during wakefulness before and after long-term (~6 months) home CPAP therapy. In order to enhance parameter estimation accuracy, the subjects were asked to track a randomized breathing pattern displayed on a monitor. The RCC and ABR gains increased approximately 3-fold after therapy in the subjects who used CPAP consistently for greater than 3 hours per night, but remained unchanged in those patients who were not compliant with therapy.[26]

c. Application of the minimal model has also been extended to subjects during sleep.[51] A bilevel pressure ventilator was used in assist mode to increase ventilatory variability in the sleeping SDB subjects. As in the aforementioned studies, both RCC and ABR gains were lower in SDB subjects. However, RCC gain did not change significantly with sleep-wake state in both SDB and control groups, whereas ABR gain increased approximately 3-fold during sleep (vs wake) in normal but remained unaffected by state changes in the SDB subjects (**Fig. 2**). These findings imply that the degree of impairment in

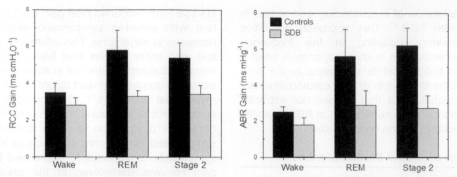

Fig. 2. Effects of SDB and sleep-wake state on the estimated impulse response magnitudes of the RCC (*left*) and ABR (*right*) components of the model. REM, rapid eye movement. (*Adapted from* Jo JA, Blasi A, Valladares E, et al. Determinants of heart rate variability in obstructive sleep apnea syndrome during wakefulness and sleep. Am J Physiol Heart Circ Physiol 2005;288:H1103–12.)

baroreflex gain in SDB is greater during sleep compared with wakefulness.

d. The minimal model has been applied to assess autonomic control in children with SDB.[52] Mean heart rate, mean blood pressure, HRV, and blood pressure variability were found to be not significantly different between SDB and control subjects. However, ABR gain was found to be almost half as large in SDB versus controls, whereas the differences in RCC gain were not significant. Change in posture from supine to standing led to significant reductions in ABR and RCC gains in both subject groups. Thus, the autonomic effects of SDB on children appear to be different from those reported in adults. Unlike the adult form, there appears to be no significant impairment of parasympathetic function in pediatric SDB, as evidenced by the relatively normal RCC impulse response.

e. Compared with age-matched normal controls, children with congenital central hypoventilation syndrome (CCHS) were found to have substantially lower overall HRV. On the other hand, there were no differences in mean heart rate, blood pressure, or blood pressure variability. Application of the minimal model led to the finding that ABR gain during supine wakefulness was almost 7-fold lower in CCHS relative to normal.[53] Orthostatic stress led to a further reduction in the ABR gain of both groups of subjects, even in CCHS subjects whose ABR gain was already low. CCHS subjects also had lower baseline RCC gains relative to normal, but in both groups, RCC gain declined with change in posture from supine to standing.

f. The minimal model has also been applied to investigate the cumulative effects of repetitive arousal alone (independent of the hypercapnia and hypoxia associated with obstructive apneas) on autonomic control.[54]

Healthy young adults were aroused from sleep by repetitive auditory stimuli over a contiguous duration of 50 minutes in stage 2 sleep. The minimal model was applied to estimate how the RCC and ABR impulse responses would change preexposure versus postexposure to the arousals. Repetitive arousal did not produce any cumulative effects on mean RRI or mean SBP. However, analysis of the data using the minimal model revealed more subtle effects. During undisturbed sleep onset, ABR gain increased with increasing depth of sleep, as had been expected. Similarly, RCC gain increased with increasing depth of sleep, although the effect was substantially greater in the LF region of the associated transfer function. However, both minimal model gains did not change significantly when sleep was interrupted by repetitive arousal. These findings suggest that exposure to repetitive arousal blocks the natural shift during normal sleep onset in sympathovagal balance toward greater vagal predominance and lower sympathetic tone.

Markers Derived from Extended Minimal Heart Rate Variability Model

The minimal HRV model has been extended to incorporate potential nonlinearities in the dynamics of the autonomic modulation of heart rate.[55] In addition to the linear RCC and ABR components displayed in Equation 1, the extended model includes (a) a nonlinear component characterizing second-order RCC dynamics, $h_{2RCC}(\tau_1, \tau_2)$; (b) a nonlinear component characterizing second-order ABR dynamics, $h_{2ABR}(\tau_1, \tau_2)$; and (c) a component describing the multiplicative interaction of the effects of respiration and blood pressure on heart rate, $h_{RCC \cdot ABR}(\tau_1, \tau_2)$. The complete mathematical formulation of this extended model is

$$\Delta RRI(t) = \sum_{\tau=0}^{P} h_{RCC}(\tau)\Delta V(t-\tau) + \sum_{\tau=0}^{P} h_{ABR}(\tau)\Delta SBP(t-\tau)$$
$$+ \sum_{\tau_1=0}^{P} \sum_{\tau_2=0}^{P} h_{2RCC}(\tau_1,\tau_2)\Delta V(t-\tau_1)\Delta V(t-\tau_2)$$
$$+ \sum_{\tau_1=0}^{P} \sum_{\tau_2=0}^{P} h_{2ABR}(\tau_1,\tau_2)\Delta SBP(t-\tau_1)\Delta SBP(t-\tau_2) \qquad (3)$$
$$+ \sum_{\tau_1=0}^{P} \sum_{\tau_2=0}^{P} h_{RCC.ABR}(\tau_1,\tau_2)\Delta V(t-\tau_1)\Delta SBP(t-\tau_2) + \varepsilon_{RRI}(t).$$

Although the nonlinear terms in Equation 3 may look abstract and formidable, each of these components has an interpretation that corresponds to observations described in the physiologic literature. The nonlinear second-order component of RCC dynamics represents the independent effect of tidal volume on RCC gain, such that as tidal volume increases at a given respiratory frequency, RCC gain increases.[56] The nonlinear second-order component of ABR dynamics represents the saturation effect on heart rate as the amplitude of the change in blood pressure increases, a well-known characteristic of baroreceptor function.[57] The "cross-kernel," $h_{RCC.ABR}(\tau_1, \tau_2)$, represents the respiratory modulation of baroreflex gain, such that a brief increase in blood pressure occurring during expiration exerts a greater effect on RRI than a similar pulse occurring during inspiration, an observation first described by Eckberg and Orshan.[58] The simplest "marker" that can be derived from these nonlinear components is the kernel magnitude, defined as the difference between maximum and minimum values of each estimated second-order kernel.

Application of the extended model to data from normals and subjects with SDB revealed significantly reduced nonlinear ABR and interaction kernel magnitudes in SDB, whereas the nonlinear RCC component was relatively unchanged. In particular, the nonlinear ABR kernel magnitude was substantially lower in SDB relative to controls. This parameter increased from wakefulness to sleep (by almost 2-fold during stage 2 sleep) in the control group, whereas it was almost unchanged in the obstructive sleep apnea syndrome group. These findings and the results from the linear ABR gains indicate that the arterial baroreflex mechanism, which becomes stronger during sleep in normals, is impaired and does not adapt accordingly during sleep in subjects with SDB.

MODEL-DERIVED MARKERS OF PERIPHERAL VASCULAR CONTROL

Although the primary focus of the studies discussed above was on the use of the minimal model to partition HRV into functional components representing RCC and baroreflex-mediated modulation, several of these studies also examined the "other half" of the closed-loop model in which respiration and changes in RRI contribute to blood pressure variability (see **Fig. 1**). RRI and stroke volume, along with total peripheral resistance, determine the value of SBP on a beat-to-beat basis. There is also some contribution from respiration through direct mechanical effects and, also possibly respiration-synchronous sympathetic activity, on stroke volume. However, a key problem is that the resulting equation for SBP variability (analogous to that for HRV as represented by Equation 1) is much harder to solve, given that some of the important auxiliary variables, for example, stroke volume and total peripheral resistance, are generally not available from the noninvasive measurements that are made in the clinical setting. On the other hand, knowledge of the interrelationships between some of these variables, for example, SBP and total peripheral resistance, could provide useful information that relates more specifically to sympathetic control of the peripheral vasculature.

Continuous Measurement of Peripheral Vascular Conductance

Although there are several methods for assessing vascular resistance, an increasingly popular tool used in the sleep laboratory is peripheral arterial tonometry (PAT), which measures the fluctuations in digit blood volume using a finger plethysmograph coupled to a constant-volume, variable pressure pneumatic system.[59] Reductions in beat-to-beat amplitude of these fluctuations reflect peripheral vasoconstriction, which is modulated by the sympathetic nervous system. Profound peripheral vasoconstriction resulting from sympathetic surges, following upper airway obstruction and arousal from sleep, constitutes the basis of using PAT for detection of OSA. By measuring peripheral vascular responsiveness at the fingertip, which has high density of α-sympathetic innervation and a high degree of blood flow rate lability, Schnall and coworkers[59] found that the blood flow patterns to be associated with apneas, thus serving as markers of the occurrence and severity of the apneas. Another study investigated the effect of upper airway obstruction and arousal on PAT in subjects with OSA.[60] The amplitude of the within-beat fluctuations in the continuous PAT signal was used as an indicator of vasoconstriction, which was reported to be associated with an increase in sympathetic nerve activity and upper airway obstruction that terminates with arousal. They found that PAT amplitude was signifi-

local factors in addition to the baroreflex control of sympathetic outflow to the peripheral vasculature. For instance, blood pressure fluctuations at the level of the finger could affect local blood flow through changes in endothelial function.[61] As well, previous reports have indicated the presence of strong respiratory modulation of muscle sympathetic nerve activity measured from peroneal nerve.[62] Moreover, a deep breath or a sigh has been reported to trigger peripheral vasoconstriction,[63,64] which further suggests a modulatory influence of respiration on G_{PV}. The authors found through a closed-loop simulation model of blood pressure variability that this sigh-vasoconstriction response cannot be reproduced without incorporating a direct respiratory modulation effect on total peripheral resistance.[65] Thus, with these considerations in mind, the following minimal model of peripheral vascular conductance has been proposed:

$$
\begin{aligned}
\Delta G_{PV}(t) = &\sum_{\tau=0}^{P} h_{RPC}(\tau)\Delta V(t-\tau) + \sum_{\tau=0}^{P} h_{BPC}(\tau)\Delta BP(t-\tau) \\
&+ \sum_{\tau_1=0}^{P}\sum_{\tau_2=0}^{P} h_{2RPC}(\tau_1,\tau_2)\Delta V(t-\tau_1)\Delta V(t-\tau_2) \\
&+ \sum_{\tau_1=0}^{P}\sum_{\tau_2=0}^{P} h_{2BPC}(\tau_1,\tau_2)\Delta BP(t-\tau_1)\Delta BP(t-\tau_2) \\
&+ \sum_{\tau_1=0}^{P}\sum_{\tau_2=0}^{P} h_{RPC.BPC}(\tau_1,\tau_2)\Delta V(t-\tau_1)\Delta BP(t-\tau_2) + \varepsilon_{GPV}(t).
\end{aligned}
\tag{4}
$$

cantly reduced as a consequence of airflow obstruction. In addition, periods of induced airflow obstruction that resulted in arousal would even further decrease the beat-to-beat amplitude of the PAT signal. Because a reduction in the amplitude of the PAT signal (PATamp) represents peripheral vasoconstriction, it would appear reasonable to use PATamp as a surrogate measure of peripheral vascular conductance, G_{PV}, the inverse of peripheral vascular resistance.

Minimal Model of Peripheral Vascular Conductance

It is well known that total peripheral resistance is modulated by sympathetically mediated changes in vascular tone driven by baroreceptor feedback generated by changes in blood pressure. Because G_{PV}, as approximated by PATamp, provides only a regional component of systemic vascular conductance, one would expect that G_{PV} is modulated by

Equation 4 is similar in structure to the extended model of HRV (as defined by Equation 3) and is shown schematically in **Fig. 3**. The left panels of **Fig. 3** display an example of the inputs, beat-to-beat pressures (BP) and respiration (ΔV), and output, beat-to-beat PATamp (taken to represent ΔG_{PV}). Changes in peripheral vascular conductance, ΔG_{PV}, are postulated to result from the linear and nonlinear quadratic effects of influences from respiration, fluctuations in blood pressure, and the interaction between these 2 inputs. In Equation 4, h_{BPC} and h_{2BPC}, respectively, represent the (linear) impulse response and nonlinear kernel of the effect of blood pressure fluctuations on ΔG_{PV}. h_{RPC} and h_{2RPC} correspond to the impulse response and nonlinear kernel characterizing the dynamics of ΔG_{PV} in response to respiration. $h_{BPC,RPC}$ represents the dynamics resulting from the interaction of blood pressure and respiration. The final term in Equation 4, ε_{GPV}, represents all extraneous influences

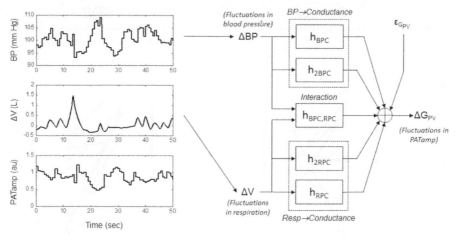

Fig. 3. (*left*) Data collected from a subject during spontaneous breathing. BP, beat-averaged arterial blood pressure; ΔV, change in lung volume (respiration); PATamp, beat-to-beat amplitude of the peripheral arterial tonometer signal. BP and ΔV are considered the inputs, and PATamp, taken to represent the change in peripheral vascular conductance (ΔG_{PV}), is treated as the output. (*right*) The linear and nonlinear components of the model (see Equation 4) are estimated from these data.

on ΔG_{PV} that cannot be explained by the model. As in the minimal model of HRV, compact descriptors are extracted from the magnitudes and shapes of the estimated impulse responses and nonlinear kernels and used as the "markers" of the autonomic mechanisms responsible for regulating peripheral vascular conductance.

Application of Minimal Model of Peripheral Vascular Conductance to Sleep-Disordered Breathing

Because the minimal model of peripheral vascular conductance is a relatively recent development, there have been fewer published applications of this methodology.[66,67] In the study of Chalacheva and Khoo,[66] obese adolescents participated in a study that included the following: (1) noninvasive measurements during wakefulness of respiratory airflow, ECG, continuous blood pressure, and PAT during supine and standing postures (10-minute recording per posture); (2) morning fasting blood samples, followed by a frequently sampled intravenous glucose tolerance test; and (3) prior night polysomnography. To investigate the combined effect of SDB and insulin resistance (IR) on autonomic reactivity due to orthostatic stress, the subjects were divided into 2 groups (controls vs SDB + IR) based on their obstructive apnea hypopnea index and insulin sensitivity. "Autonomic reactivity" was quantified as the change in BPC or RPC gains from supine to standing. Overall, the linear and nonlinear gains derived from the minimal model decreased from supine to standing. The SDB + IR group displayed markedly larger

reductions in BPC linear and nonlinear gains from supine to standing compared with the control subjects. **Fig. 4** displays how the nonlinear BPC gain changed with orthostatic stress on an individual subject-by-subject basis as well as on a group basis (controls vs SDB + IR). Thus, in the SDB + IR subjects, there was a substantially larger reduction in the nonlinear contribution to baroreflex gain due to change in posture from supine to standing. The physiologic basis of this difference in orthostatic response remains unclear at this point, but the ability of the minimal model to detect this difference in response between the subject groups suggests the possibility of using model-derived markers to monitor the progression of autonomic dysfunction in individual subjects with SDB and/or metabolic syndrome.

SURROGATE OF CONTINUOUS BLOOD PRESSURE

An important limitation on the practical utility of using the aforementioned minimal models is the need for noninvasive measurement of continuous blood pressure, which is highly expensive and thus problematic for deployment in large-scale clinical studies. On the other hand, pulse plethysmography is routinely measured. The speed at which the arterial pressure pulse travels is directly proportional to blood pressure, assuming constant elasticity of the arterial wall. Although pulse transit time (PTT) is not a reliable predictor of SBP, there is a good correlation between beat-to-beat fluctuations in PTT (PTTV) and the variability in SBP.[68] The authors have taken advantage of this observation to

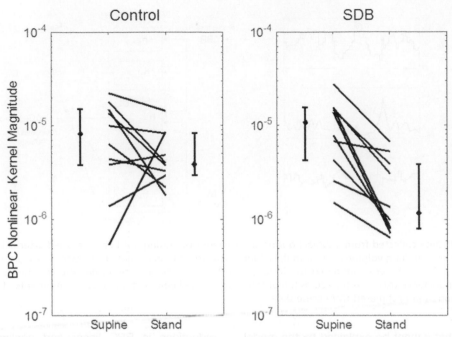

Fig. 4. Autonomic reactivity to orthostatic stress in obese adolescents with SDB and IR versus obese adolescent controls. The model-derived marker shown here is the magnitude of the blood pressure to peripheral vascular conductance nonlinear kernel. BPC nonlinear gain decreased significantly more in SDB subjects compared with controls following change in posture from supine to standing. Lines connect the supine and standing values of each individual. Closed circles and error bars represent group medians and interquartile ranges of the parameter estimates.

introduce a surrogate measure of baroreflex gain, BRS_{PTT}, that is derived from HRV and PTTV, and have demonstrated that BRS_{PTT} correlates robustly with corresponding measures of baroreflex gain derived from noninvasive continuous measurement of arterial blood pressure.[69] BRS_{PTT} provides information that complements the results derived from HRV alone; in particular, this index provides an indication as to whether the detected differences in HRV could be the result of alterations in baroreflex function. Since the baroreceptors continuously inhibit sympathetic efferent activity, depressed BRS_{PTT} can indicate sympathetic overactivity. Using data derived from polysomnograms in a large-scale study of sleep apnea, the authors found that BRS_{PTT} is correlated with measures of impaired glucose tolerance, in subjects with or without SDB.[70] This association suggests that these low-cost, noninvasively derived autonomic indices may be useful in practice as biomarkers of abnormal glucose metabolism or autonomic dysfunction.

SUMMARY

In this article, the authors have presented a comprehensive, but nevertheless incomplete, overview of the long-term effects of SDB on cardiovascular autonomic function in humans, focusing directly on the knowledge derived from continuous measurements of heart rate, blood pressure, and respiration obtained noninvasively during wakefulness and sleep. The rapid development of new and low-cost wearable technologies presages the need for smarter utilization and improved methods for interpreting the ever-increasing amounts of physiologic data being collected by these devices. Conventional univariate analyses of heart rate, blood pressure, and respiratory variability provide useful information about cardiovascular autonomic control. However, a multivariate model-based approach, by elucidating the causal, dynamic interrelationships among these measurements, provides the ability to interpret the data on a more contextual basis and thus make inferences that are more accurate and relevant to autonomic health.

ACKNOWLEDGMENTS

The work reported in this article was funded in part by the US National Institutes of Health grants HL090451, HL077785, EB001978, and HL105210.

REFERENCES

1. Leung RS, Bradley TD. Sleep apnea and cardiovascular disease. Am J Respir Crit Care Med 2001; 164(12):2147–65.

2. Caples SM, Garcia-Touchard A, Somers VK. Sleep-disordered breathing and cardiovascular risk. Sleep 2007;30(3):291–303. Available at: http://www.ncbi.nlm.nih.gov/pubmed/17425225. Accessed April 19, 2016.

3. Peppard PE, Young T, Palta M, et al. Prospective study of the association between sleep-disordered breathing and hypertension. N Engl J Med 2000; 342(19):1378–84.

4. Shahar E, Whitney CW, Redline S, et al. Sleep-disordered breathing and cardiovascular disease: cross-sectional results of the Sleep Heart Health Study. Am J Respir Crit Care Med 2001;163(1): 19–25.

5. Nieto FJ, Young TB, Lind BK, et al. Association of sleep-disordered breathing, sleep apnea, and hypertension in a large community-based study. Sleep Heart Health Study. JAMA 2000;283(14):1829–36. Available at: http://www.ncbi.nlm.nih.gov/pubmed/10770144. Accessed April 19, 2016..

6. Schaub CG, Schneider H, O'Donnell CP. Mechanisms of acute and chronic blood pressure elevation in animal models of obstructive sleep apnea. In: Bradley TD, Floras JS, editors. Sleep apnea: implications in cardiovascular and cerebrovascular disease 2. New York: Marcel Dekker; 2000. p. 159–79.

7. Brooks D, Horner RL, Kozar LF, et al. Obstructive sleep apnea as a cause of systemic hypertension. Evidence from a canine model. J Clin Invest 1997; 99(1):106–9.

8. Fletcher EC, Lesske J, Behm R, et al. Carotid chemoreceptors, systemic blood pressure, and chronic episodic hypoxia mimicking sleep apnea. J Appl Physiol 1992;72(5):1978–84. Available at: http://www.ncbi.nlm.nih.gov/pubmed/1601808.

9. Fletcher EC, Lesske J, Culman J, et al. Sympathetic denervation blocks blood pressure elevation in episodic hypoxia. Hypertension 1992;20(5):612–9. Available at: http://www.ncbi.nlm.nih.gov/pubmed/1428112. Accessed April 19, 2016..

10. Weiss JW, Liu MDY, Huang J. Physiological basis for a causal relationship of obstructive sleep apnoea to hypertension. Exp Physiol 2007;92(1):21–6.

11. Leung RST. Sleep-disordered breathing: autonomic mechanisms and arrhythmias. Prog Cardiovasc Dis 2009;51(4):324–38.

12. Carlson JT, Hedner J, Elam M, et al. Augmented resting sympathetic activity in awake patients with obstructive sleep apnea. Chest 1993;103(6): 1763–8. Available at: http://www.ncbi.nlm.nih.gov/pubmed/8404098.

13. Somers VK, Dyken ME, Clary MP, et al. Sympathetic neural mechanisms in obstructive sleep apnea. J Clin Invest 1995;96(4):1897–904.

14. Narkiewicz K, van de Borne PJ, Cooley RL, et al. Sympathetic activity in obese subjects with and without obstructive sleep apnea. Circulation 1998; 98(8):772–6. Available at: http://www.ncbi.nlm.nih.gov/pubmed/9727547. Accessed April 19, 2016.

15. Waradekar NV, Sinoway LI, Zwillich CW, et al. Influence of treatment on muscle sympathetic nerve activity in sleep apnea. Am J Respir Crit Care Med 1996;153(4 Pt 1):1333–8.

16. Hedner J, Darpö B, Ejnell H, et al. Reduction in sympathetic activity after long-term CPAP treatment in sleep apnoea: cardiovascular implications. Eur Respir J 1995;8(2):222–9. Available at: http://www.ncbi.nlm.nih.gov/pubmed/7758555. Accessed April 19, 2016.

17. Narkiewicz K, Kato M, Phillips BG, et al. Nocturnal continuous positive airway pressure decreases daytime sympathetic traffic in obstructive sleep apnea. Circulation 1999;100(23):2332–5. Available at: http://www.ncbi.nlm.nih.gov/pubmed/10587337.

18. Imadojemu VA, Mawji Z, Kunselman A, et al. Sympathetic chemoreflex responses in obstructive sleep apnea and effects of continuous positive airway pressure therapy. Chest 2007;131(5):1406–13.

19. Xie A, Skatrud JB, Crabtree DC, et al. Neurocirculatory consequences of intermittent asphyxia in humans. J Appl Physiol 2000;89(4):1333–9. Available at: http://www.ncbi.nlm.nih.gov/pubmed/11007566.

20. Cutler MJ, Swift NM, Keller DM, et al. Hypoxia-mediated prolonged elevation of sympathetic nerve activity after periods of intermittent hypoxic apnea. J Appl Physiol 2004;96(2):754–61.

21. Leuenberger UA, Brubaker D, Quraishi SA, et al. Effects of intermittent hypoxia on sympathetic activity and blood pressure in humans. Auton Neurosci 2005;121(1–2):87–93.

22. Leuenberger UA, Hogeman CS, Quraishi SA, et al. Short-term intermittent hypoxia enhances sympathetic responses to continuous hypoxia in humans. J Appl Physiol 2007;103(3):835–42.

23. Lai CJ, Yang CC, Hsu YY, et al. Enhanced sympathetic outflow and decreased baroreflex sensitivity are associated with intermittent hypoxia-induced systemic hypertension in conscious rats. J Appl Physiol 2006;100(6):1974–82.

24. Narkiewicz K, Pesek CA, Kato M, et al. Baroreflex control of sympathetic nerve activity and heart rate in obstructive sleep apnea. Hypertension 1998; 32(6):1039–43. Available at: http://www.ncbi.nlm.nih.gov/pubmed/9856970. Accessed April 19, 2016.

25. Belozeroff V, Berry RB, Khoo MC. Model-based assessment of autonomic control in obstructive sleep apnea syndrome. Sleep 2003;26(1):65–73.

26. Belozeroff V, Berry RB, Sassoon CS, et al. Effects of CPAP therapy on cardiovascular variability in obstructive sleep apnea: a closed-loop analysis. Am J Physiol Heart Circ Physiol 2002;282(1):H110–21. Available at: http://www.ncbi.nlm.nih.gov/pubmed/11748054.

27. Wallin BG, Fagius J. Peripheral sympathetic neural activity in conscious humans. Annu Rev Physiol 1988;50:565–76.

28. Mancia G, Daffonchio A, Di Rienzo M, et al. Methods to quantify sympathetic cardiovascular influences. Eur Heart J 1998;19(Suppl F):F7–13. Available at: http://www.ncbi.nlm.nih.gov/pubmed/9651729. Accessed April 19, 2016.

29. Veale D, Pépin JL, Lévy PA. Autonomic stress tests in obstructive sleep apnea syndrome and snoring. Sleep 1992;15(6):505–13. Available at: http://www.ncbi.nlm.nih.gov/pubmed/1475565. Accessed April 19, 2016.

30. Heart rate variability: standards of measurement, physiological interpretation and clinical use. Task Force of the European Society of Cardiology and the North American Society of Pacing and Electrophysiology. Circulation 1996;93(5):1043–65. Available at: http://www.ncbi.nlm.nih.gov/pubmed/8598068. Accessed April 19, 2016.

31. Eckberg DL. Sympathovagal balance: a critical appraisal. Circulation 1997;96(9):3224–32. Available at: http://www.ncbi.nlm.nih.gov/pubmed/9386196. Accessed January 14, 2015..

32. Malliani A, Pagani M, Lombardi F, et al. Cardiovascular neural regulation explored in the frequency domain. Circulation 1991;84(2):482–92. Available at: http://www.ncbi.nlm.nih.gov/pubmed/1860193. Accessed April 19, 2016.

33. Katona PG, Jih F. Respiratory sinus arrhythmia: noninvasive measure of parasympathetic cardiac control. J Appl Physiol 1975;39(5):801–5. Available at: http://www.ncbi.nlm.nih.gov/pubmed/1184518. Accessed April 19, 2016.

34. Brown TE, Beightol LA, Koh J, et al. Important influence of respiration on human R-R interval power spectra is largely ignored. J Appl Physiol 1993;75:2310–7.

35. Khoo MC, Kim TS, Berry RB. Spectral indices of cardiac autonomic function in obstructive sleep apnea. Sleep 1999;22(4):443–51. Available at: http://www.ncbi.nlm.nih.gov/pubmed/10389220. Accessed April 19, 2016.

36. Parati G, Di Rienzo M, Mancia G. How to measure baroreflex sensitivity: from the cardiovascular laboratory to daily life. J Hypertens 2000;18(1):7–19. Available at: http://www.ncbi.nlm.nih.gov/pubmed/10678538.

37. Barbieri R, Waldmann RA, Di Virgilio V, et al. Continuous quantification of baroreflex and respiratory control of heart rate by use of bivariate autoregressive techniques. Ann Noninvasive Electrocardiol 1996;1(3):264–77.

38. Eckberg DL. Respiratory sinus arrhythmia and other human cardiovascular neural periodicities. In: Dempsey JA, Pack AI, editors. Regulation of breathing. 2nd edition. New York: Marcel Dekker; 1995. p. 669–740.

39. Khoo MCK. Physiological control systems: analysis, simulation and estimation. Piscataway (NJ): Wiley/IEEE Press; 2000.

40. Marmarelis VZ. Identification of nonlinear biological systems using Laguerre expansions of kernels. Ann Biomed Eng 1993;21(6):573–89. Available at: http://www.ncbi.nlm.nih.gov/pubmed/8116911.

41. Asyali MH, Juusola M. Use of Meixner functions in estimation of Volterra kernels of nonlinear systems with delay. IEEE Trans Biomed Eng 2005;52(2):229–37.

42. Chaicharn J, Lin Z, Chen ML, et al. Model-based assessment of cardiovascular autonomic control in children with obstructive sleep apnea. Sleep 2009;32(7):927–38. Available at: http://www.ncbi.nlm.nih.gov/pubmed/19639756.

43. Baselli G, Cerutti S, Civardi S, et al. Cardiovascular variability signals: towards the identification of a closed-loop model of the neural control mechanisms. IEEE Trans Biomed Eng 1988;35(12):1033–46.

44. Mukkamala R, Mathias JM, Mullen TJ, et al. System identification of closed-loop cardiovascular control mechanisms: diabetic autonomic neuropathy. Am J Physiol 1999;276(3 Pt 2):R905–12. Available at: http://www.ncbi.nlm.nih.gov/pubmed/10070154.

45. Lucini D, Porta A, Milani O, et al. Assessment of arterial and cardiopulmonary baroreflex gains from simultaneous recordings of spontaneous cardiovascular and respiratory variability. J Hypertens 2000;18(3):281–6. Available at: http://www.ncbi.nlm.nih.gov/pubmed/10726714. Accessed April 19, 2016.

46. Thomas RJ, Mietus JE, Peng C-K, et al. An electrocardiogram-based technique to assess cardiopulmonary coupling during sleep. Sleep 2005;28(9):1151–61. Available at: http://www.ncbi.nlm.nih.gov/pubmed/16268385. Accessed July 17, 2016.

47. Thomas RJ, Weiss MD, Mietus JE, et al. Prevalent hypertension and stroke in the Sleep Heart Health Study: association with an ECG-derived spectrographic marker of cardiopulmonary coupling. Sleep 2009;32(7):897–904. Available at: http://www.pubmedcentral.nih.gov/articlerender.fcgi?artid=2706909&tool=pmcentrez&rendertype=abstract. Accessed July 17, 2016.

48. Bristow JD, Honour AJ, Pickering GW, et al. Diminished baroreflex sensitivity in high blood pressure. Circulation 1969;39(1):48–54.

49. Francis DP, Coats AJS, Ponikowski P. Chemoreflex-baroreflex interactions in cardiovascular disease. In: Bradley TD, Floras JS, editors. Sleep apnea: implications in cardiovascular and cerebrovascular disease. New York: Marcel Dekker; 2000. p. 33–60.

50. La Rovere MT, Bigger JT, Marcus FI, et al. Baroreflex sensitivity and heart-rate variability in prediction of

total cardiac mortality after myocardial infarction. Lancet 1998;351:478–84.

51. Jo JA, Blasi A, Valladares E, et al. Model-based assessment of autonomic control in obstructive sleep apnea syndrome during sleep. Am J Respir Crit Care Med 2003;167(2):128–36.

52. Lin Z, K Khoo M, Chen M, et al. Noninvasive assessment of cardiovascular autonomic control in pediatric obstructive sleep apnea syndrome. Conf Proc IEEE Eng Med Biol Soc 2005;1:776–9.

53. Lin Z, Chen ML, Keens TG, et al. Noninvasive assessment of cardiovascular autonomic control in congenital central hypoventilation syndrome. Conf Proc IEEE Eng Med Biol Soc 2004;5:3870–3.

54. Chaicharn J, Carrington M, Trinder J, et al. The effects on cardiovascular autonomic control of repetitive arousal from sleep. Sleep 2008;31(1):93–103. Available at: http://www.ncbi.nlm.nih.gov/pubmed/18220082.

55. Jo JA, Blasi A, Valladares EM, et al. A nonlinear model of cardiac autonomic control in obstructive sleep apnea syndrome. Ann Biomed Eng 2007; 35(8):1425–43.

56. Hirsch JA, Bishop B. Respiratory sinus arrhythmia in humans: how breathing pattern modulates heart rate. Am J Physiol 1981;241(4):H620–9. Available at: http://www.ncbi.nlm.nih.gov/pubmed/7315987. Accessed April 29, 2016.

57. Mancia G, Mark AL. Arterial baroreflexes in humans. In: Shepherd JT, Abboud FM, editors. Compr Physiol 2011, Supplement 8: Handbook of physiology, the cardiovascular system, peripheral circulation and organ blood flow. Bethesda (MD): American Physiological Society; 1983. p. 755–93. Available at: http://www.comprehensivephysiology.com/Wiley CDA/CompPhysArticle/refId-cp020320.html. Accessed April 29, 2016.

58. Eckberg DL, Orshan CR. Respiratory and baroreceptor reflex interactions in man. J Clin Invest 1977;59(5):780–5.

59. Schnall RP, Shlitner A, Sheffy J, et al. Periodic, profound peripheral vasoconstriction–a new marker of obstructive sleep apnea. Sleep 1999;22(7):939–46. Available at: http://www.ncbi.nlm.nih.gov/pubmed/10566912.

60. O'Donnell CP, Allan L, Atkinson P, et al. The effect of upper airway obstruction and arousal on peripheral arterial tonometry in obstructive sleep apnea. Am J

Respir Crit Care Med 2002;166(7):965–71. Available at: http://www.ncbi.nlm.nih.gov/pubmed/12359655.

61. Secomb TW. Theoretical models for regulation of blood flow. Microcirculation 2008;15(8):765–75.

62. Seals DR, Suwarno NO, Joyner MJ, et al. Respiratory modulation of muscle sympathetic nerve activity in intact and lung denervated humans. Circ Res 1993;72(2):440–54. Available at: http://www.ncbi.nlm.nih.gov/pubmed/8418993. Accessed April 29, 2016.

63. Bolton B, Carmichael EA, Sturup G. Vaso-constriction following deep inspiration. J Physiol 1936;86(1):83–94. Available at: http://www.ncbi.nlm.nih.gov/pubmed/16994738.

64. Sangkatumvong S, Khoo MCK, Kato R, et al. Peripheral vasoconstriction and abnormal parasympathetic response to sighs and transient hypoxia in sickle cell disease. Am J Respir Crit Care Med 2011;184:474–81.

65. Chalacheva P, Khoo MCK. An extended model of blood pressure variability: incorporating the respiratory modulation of vascular resistance. Conf Proc IEEE Eng Med Biol Soc 2013;2013:3825–8.

66. Chalacheva P, Khoo MCK. Estimating the baroreflex and respiratory modulation of peripheral vascular resistance. Conf Proc IEEE Eng Med Biol Soc 2014;2014:2936–9.

67. Chalacheva P, Kato RM, Sangkatumvong S, et al. Autonomic responses to cold face stimulation in sickle cell disease: a time-varying model analysis. Physiol Rep 2015;3(7). http://dx.doi.org/10.14814/phy2.12463.

68. Payne RA, Symeonides CN, Webb DJ, et al. Pulse transit time measured from the ECG: an unreliable marker of beat-to-beat blood pressure. J Appl Physiol 2006;100(1):136–41.

69. Khoo MCK, Wang W, Chalacheva P. Monitoring ultradian changes in cardiorespiratory control in obstructive sleep apnea syndrome. Conf Proc IEEE Eng Med Biol Soc 2011;2011:1487–90.

70. Wang W, Redline S, Khoo MCK. Autonomic markers of impaired glucose metabolism: effects of sleep-disordered breathing. J Diabetes Sci Technol 2012;6(5):1159–71. Available at: http://www.pubmedcentral.nih.gov/articlerender.fcgi?artid=3570851&tool=pmcentrez&rendertype=abstract. Accessed April 29, 2016.

Adverse Effects of Psychotropic Medications on Sleep

Karl Doghramji, MD[a],*, William C. Jangro, DO[b]

KEYWORDS

- Antidepressant • Antipsychotic • Insomnia • Sedation • Adverse effects • Sleep • Somnolence

KEY POINTS

- Psychotropic medications have a broad range of mechanisms of action, which are presumed to be involved in their sleep-related adverse effects.
- Insomnia and daytime somnolence are common adverse effects of these medications.
- These effects can be beneficial or detrimental depending on the particular symptoms of the patient's psychiatric disorder.
- Being aware of an agent's most likely adverse effects on sleep can aid the prescriber in choosing an agent that is more likely to improve the sleep component of a patient's psychiatric disorder.

ANTIDEPRESSANTS

People suffering from depressive disorders typically complain of difficulty falling asleep, frequent awakenings, early morning wakening, and non-refreshing sleep. Polysomnographic studies of depressed persons have confirmed these findings and show reduced rapid eye movement (REM) latency, increased REMs, increased total time in REM sleep, reduced slow wave sleep (SWS), and frequent awakenings throughout the night.[1] Antidepressants are widely prescribed for mood and anxiety disorders. According to the National Health and Nutrition Examination Survey, 11% of Americans over the age of 12 are taking an antidepressant medication.[2] Most of these antidepressant medications are thought to exert their effects through modulation of various monoamines as well as interactions with receptors such as histamine and muscarinic cholinergic receptors. Through these interactions, antidepressants can have a significant impact on sleep physiology. The central processes governing sleep and wakefulness are dependent on the complex interaction of these various neurotransmitter systems.[3,4] The ascending arousal system, which traverses from the brainstem regions to the cerebral cortex, consists of noradrenergic neurons of the ventrolateral medulla and locus coeruleus, cholinergic neurons in the pedunculopontine and laterodorsal tegmental nuclei, serotonergic neurons in the dorsal raphe nucleus, dopaminergic neurons of the ventral periaqueductal gray matter, and histaminergic neurons of the tuberomammillary nucleus. Orexin (hypocretin) neurons of the lateral hypothalamic area contribute as well and

This article originally appeared in *Psychiatric Clinics of North America*, Volume 39, Issue 3, September 2016.
Dr K. Doghramji owns stock in Merck and is a consultant for Merck, Inspire, Jazz, Xenoport, Teva, Pfizer, and Pernix. Dr W. C. Jangro has nothing to disclose.
[a] Fellowship in Sleep Medicine, Department of Psychiatry and Human Behavior, Jefferson Sleep Disorders Center, Sidney Kimmel Medical College, Thomas Jefferson University, Walnut Towers, 5th Floor, 211 South 9th Street, Philadelphia, PA 19107, USA; [b] Adult Residency Training Program, Department of Psychiatry and Human Behavior, Sidney Kimmel Medical College, Thomas Jefferson University, 833 Chestnut Street, Suite 210, Philadelphia, PA 19107, USA
* Corresponding author.
E-mail address: karl.doghramji@jefferson.edu

Abbreviations

5-HT	5-Hydroxytryptamine
ADHD	Attention-deficit/hyperactivity disorder
H1	Histamine 1 receptor
MAOI	Monoamine oxidase inhibitor
MDD	Major depressive disorder
NNTH	Numbers needed to treat to harm
PLM	Periodic limb movement
PSG	Polysomnogram
PSQI	Pittsburgh Sleep Quality Index
REM	Rapid eye movement
RLS	Restless legs syndrome
SNRI	Serotonin-norepinephrine reuptake inhibitor
SOL	Sleep onset latency
SRED	Sleep-related eating disorders
SSRI	Selective serotonin reuptake inhibitor
SWS	Slow wave sleep
TCA	Tricyclic antidepressant
TST	Total sleep time
VLPO	Ventrolateral preoptic nucleus
WASO	Wakefulness after sleep onset

are thought to have a modulatory influence on the transition between sleep and wakefulness. On the other hand, the sleep system is thought to be controlled by activation of sleep-active cells in the ventrolateral preoptic nucleus (VLPO), which contain the inhibitory neurotransmitters γ-aminobutyric acid and galanin. These cells project to the essential components of the ascending arousal system. Inhibition of the arousal system by the VLPO during sleep is critical for the maintenance and consolidation of sleep.

Antidepressant classes and their receptor profiles are listed in **Table 1**. For definitions of

polysomnographic terms, readers are referred to standard scoring manuals.[5]

SELECTIVE SEROTONIN REUPTAKE INHIBITORS
Subjective Effects

Subjective complaints of insomnia and daytime somnolence are common in people with depression being treated with selective serotonin reuptake inhibitors (SSRIs). Of the SSRIs currently indicated for the treatment of depression, fluoxetine's effects on sleep have been the most thoroughly studied. These effects may represent a class effect. Fluoxetine has been found to cause both significant activation and sedation compared with placebo.[6] Rates of activation tend to be stable at dosages between 5 and 40 mg per day, but increase at dosages greater than 40 mg per day. On the other hand, sedation increases linearly up to dosages of 40 mg per day and then remains stable at dosages between 40 and 60 mg per day. Rates of subjectively reported insomnia and daytime somnolence for various SSRIs are noted in **Fig. 1**.

Polysomnographic Effects

Fluoxetine can cause a decrease in sleep continuity as well as other polysomnographic effects, including REM suppression,[7–10] decreased sleep efficiency,[3,6,11] and increased number of awakenings.[4,7] Disruption in sleep continuity has been found to correlate with plasma levels of fluoxetine and its biologically active metabolite, norfluoxetine. Thus, changes in sleep continuity may develop over time as plasma levels increase because of accumulation of the drug.[3] Fluoxetine

Table 1
Antidepressant classes and their sleep-related pharmacologic profiles

Medication/Class	Sleep-related Pharmacology	Effects on Sleep Architecture
SSRI	5-HT reuptake inhibition	REM suppression, increased REM latency
SNRI	5-HT, norepinephrine reuptake inhibition	REM suppression, increased REM latency
Trazodone/ nefazodone	5-HT 2 antagonism	Decreased sleep latency, increased SWS
Mirtazapine	5-HT 2 antagonism, H1 antagonism	Decreased sleep latency, increased SWS
TCA	5-HT, norepinephrine reuptake inhibition, H1 antagonism	Decreased sleep latency, REM suppression, increased REM latency

Adapted from Barkoukis TR, Matheson JK, Ferber R, et al, editors. Therapy in sleep medicine. Philadelphia: Elsevier Saunders; 2012.

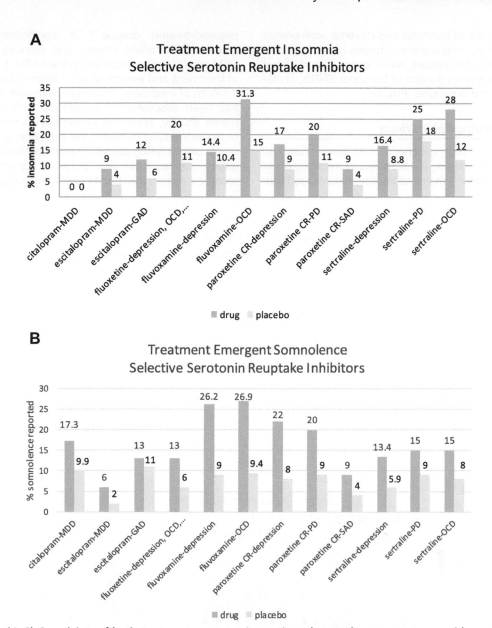

Fig. 1. (*A*, *B*) Complaints of both treatment emergent insomnia and somnolence are common with most SSRIs. Where rates are reported as 0%, the event occurred in less than 2% of patients treated with the medication and at rates less than that with placebo. Caution should be taken in using these figures to predict the incidence of adverse effects in usual clinical practice where conditions and patient characteristics may differ from those in the respective clinical trials. In addition, results are not strictly comparative because they are derived from separate studies performed under differing conditions and with different methodologies. (*Data from* US Food and Drug Administration. FDA Approved Drug Products. Available at: http://www.accessdata.fda.gov/scripts/cder/drugsatfda/index.cfm. Accessed October 2, 2015.)

also increases the number of oculomotor movements during non-rapid eye movement sleep.[12–14] Although this has not been a consistent finding, it may suggest a generalized increase in central arousal.[15]

SEROTONIN-NOREPINEPHRINE REUPTAKE INHIBITORS
Subjective Effects

Serotonin-norepinephrine reuptake inhibitors (SNRIs) are associated with frequent subjective complaints of insomnia and daytime somnolence as well as vivid dreams. Studies using polysomnography techniques have been limited. Most studies involve the use of the older SNRIs, venlafaxine and duloxetine (**Fig. 2**).

Polysomnographic Effects

Treatment with venlafaxine has been shown to cause an increase in wakefulness after sleep onset (WASO) after 1 month of treatment compared with placebo-treated groups.[16] It significantly increases REM onset latency and reduces total REM time. These effects are evident after 1 week of treatment and persist when monitored for after 1 month of treatment. Treatment with venlafaxine has been associated with periodic limb movements (PLMs), repetitive involuntary movements of the extremities, typically the legs, during sleep or just before falling asleep. These repetitive involuntary movements are polysomnographically recorded as periodic bursts of electromyographic

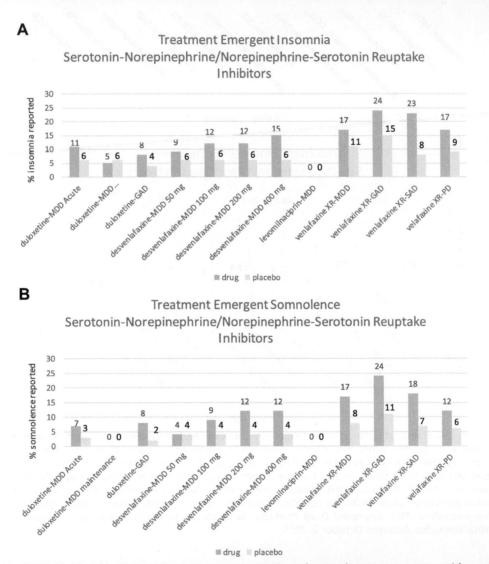

Fig. 2. (*A, B*) Complaints of both treatment emergent insomnia and somnolence are common with most SSRIs/SNRIs. Where rates are reported as 0%, the event occurred in less than 2% of patients treated with the medication and at rates less than that with placebo. Caution should be taken in using these figures to predict the incidence of adverse effects in usual clinical practice where conditions and patient characteristics may differ from those in the respective clinical trials. In addition, results are not strictly comparative because they are derived from separate studies performed under differing conditions and with different methodologies. (*Data from* US Food and Drug Administration. FDA Approved Drug Products. Available at: http://www.accessdata.fda.gov/scripts/cder/drugsatfda/index.cfm. Accessed October 2, 2015.)

activity in the anterior tibialis electrodes of the lower extremities. The pathophysiologic basis of for these movements is unknown, and the basis of the effects of venlafaxine in promoting these movements is also unknown. Effects can be continuous and worsen over time, with rates of greater than 25 PLMs per hour being reported.[17] In some, these movements may persist for up to a week after discontinuation of treatment.

Trazodone

Trazodone's use as an antidepressant is often limited by its tendency to produce daytime somnolence. In that respect, it is often used, at low doses, as a sleep aid or coadministered with an SSRI to decrease the SSRIs' deleterious and disruptive effects on sleep. This effect has not been well studied. When administered alone to depressed patients, trazodone has been shown to increase total sleep time (TST), decrease sleep onset latency (SOL), reduce WASO, increase SWS, and increase REM latency.[18]

Mirtazapine

Daytime somnolence is a common adverse effect of mirtazapine. In clinical trials, up to 54% of patients treated with mirtazapine reported it as an adverse event.[19] However, in practice, this effect can be used to improve sleep disturbances in select populations, although this effect has not been well explored. Mirtazapine produces predominantly antihistaminergic effects at lower doses, compared with increasingly predominant noradrenergic effects at higher doses.[20] Because of this unique pharmacologic profile, mirtazapine is thought to produce relatively more sedation at doses less than 30 mg per day.[21] In depressed patients, it has been shown to significantly increase TST and sleep efficiency and significantly reduce SOL, without significantly altering REM sleep parameters.[22] Although mirtazapine has typically been associated with beneficial effects on sleep, disturbing dreams and confusional states were reported during clinical trials.[23]

Bupropion

Bupropion is associated with reports of insomnia in patients treated for depression and seasonal affective disorder with rates ranging from 11% to 20% depending on the dose, formulation, and condition being treated. However, electroencephalogram studies have shown bupropion to be one of the few antidepressants that actually shortens REM latency and increases total REM sleep time.[24] This finding is in contrast to most other antidepressants, which are prominent suppressants of REM sleep.

New antidepressants

Several medications have recently been approved for the treatment of major depressive disorder (MDD). These medications include levomilnacipran (2013), vilazodone (2011), and vortioxetine (2013). Sleep disturbance was not listed as a common adverse effect in clinical studies for levomilnacipran.[25] Somnolence, insomnia, and abnormal dreams were listed as common adverse effects in clinical trials with vilazodone.[26] Abnormal dreams, but not insomnia or somnolence, were listed as a common adverse effect in clinical trials with vortioxetine.[27] Further studies, including polysomnographic testing in patients taking these medications, are needed to better understand the effects of these newer agents on sleep (Fig. 3).

TRICYCLIC ANTIDEPRESSANTS
Subjective Effects

Tertiary amine tricyclic antidepressants (TCAs; amitriptyline, trimipramine) tend to be more sedating, whereas secondary amine TCAs (desipramine, nortriptyline) tend to be more activating. Therefore, it may easier to choose a particular agent in this class that will have the desired effect on sleep profile compared with other classes of antidepressants. Sedating, tertiary amine TCAs tend to shorten SOL, improve sleep continuity and efficiency, and reduce WASO.[28–30] Activating, secondary amine TCAs, on the other hand, tend to prolong SOL, reduce sleep efficiency, and increase WASO.[31] The TCA doxepin, first approved in 1969 for the management of major depression and anxiety and as a topical preparation (5% cream) for pruritus, was recently reformulated in lower oral doses (3 mg and 6 mg) with demonstrated efficacy for insomnia characterized by difficulties with sleep maintenance following sleep onset.[32] In addition to subjective improvements in insomnia measures, polysomnographic measures of wake after sleep onset, TST, and sleep efficiency have been shown to improve following its administration at bedtime. Although its mechanism of action is not known, it is presumed to promote sleep by antagonizing the histamine-based arousal pathways.[33,34]

Polysomnographic Effects

All TCAs, with the exception of trimipramine, suppress REM sleep; this is manifested by an increase in REM latency and a decreased percentage of time spent in REM sleep.[35–37] At standard antidepressant doses, clomipramine appears to have the most potent REM suppressant effects, although comparative data are limited. Placebo and plasma concentration-controlled studies of maintenance

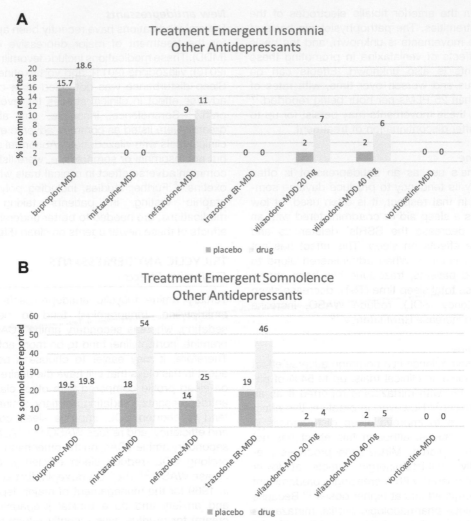

Fig. 3. (*A*, *B*) Complaints of both treatment emergent insomnia and somnolence are common with most antidepressants. Where rates are reported as 0%, the event occurred in less than 2% of patients treated with the medication and at rates less than that with placebo. Caution should be taken in using these figures to predict the incidence of adverse effects in usual clinical practice where conditions and patient characteristics may differ from those in the respective clinical trials. In addition, results are not strictly comparative because they are derived from separate studies performed under differing conditions and with different methodologies. (*Data from* US Food and Drug Administration. FDA Approved Drug Products. Available at: http://www.accessdata.fda.gov/scripts/cder/drugsatfda/index.cfm. Accessed October 2, 2015.)

nortriptyline therapy in depressed elderly patients have shown that REM suppression and increased REM latency persist, even in those with no recurrence of depression in 1 year.[38,39] In addition, patients on TCA therapy tend to report intense, vivid dreams, and even nightmares. Recall of dreams may be due to the REM-suppressing effect of the TCA leading to increased pressure for REM.

Monoamine oxidase inhibitors

Treatment with monoamine oxidase inhibitors (MAOIs) is associated with frequent complaints

of insomnia, especially with tranylcypromine, which is structurally similar to amphetamine and is more stimulating. MAOIs tend to cause prolonged SOL, impaired sleep continuity, and increased WASO.[40,41] REM suppression is also common, possibly more so with irreversible MAOIs than with reversible MAOIs like moclobemide.[42] REM suppression typically occurs quickly after initiation and persists for months if the medication is continued. REM rebound occurs with discontinuation of therapy and can lead to intense and vivid dreams (**Fig. 4**).

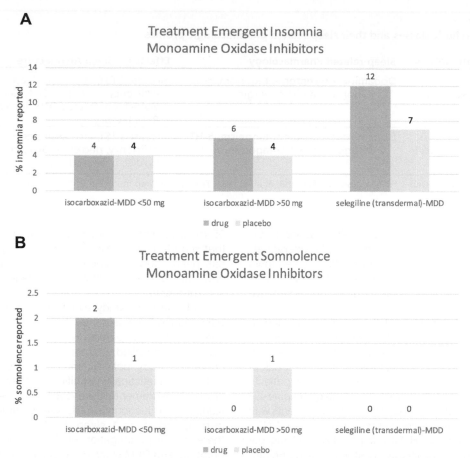

Fig. 4. (*A*, *B*) Complaints of both treatment emergent insomnia and somnolence are common with most MAOIs. Where rates are reported as 0%, the event occurred in less than 2% of patients treated with the medication and at rates less than that with placebo. Caution should be taken in using these figures to predict the incidence of adverse effects in usual clinical practice where conditions and patient characteristics may differ from those in the respective clinical trials. In addition, results are not strictly comparative because they are derived from separate studies performed under differing conditions and with different methodologies. (*Data from* US Food and Drug Administration. FDA Approved Drug Products. Available at: http://www.accessdata.fda.gov/scripts/cder/drugsatfda/index.cfm. Accessed October 2, 2015.)

ANTIPSYCHOTICS

Antipsychotics are indicated for the treatment of schizophrenia and other psychotic disorders. Many of the atypical antipsychotics also have indications for the treatment of bipolar disorder and adjunctive treatment of MDDs. Daytime somnolence and sedation seem to be a much more common problem with antipsychotics compared with insomnia. Antipsychotics are thought to exert much of their indicated effects through antagonism of dopamine receptors. Many typical and atypical antipsychotics also exert effects on various monoamines as well as histamine and muscarinic cholinergic receptors. These effects may increase the likelihood of somnolence and can also alter certain polysomnogram (PSG) sleep parameters (**Table 2**).

Typical Antipsychotics

Studies evaluating the effects of typical antipsychotic drugs in patients with schizophrenia are limited. Of the studies that are available,[43–45] haloperidol, thiothixene, and flupentixol possibly reduce stage 2 sleep latency, increase TST and sleep efficiency, and significantly increase REM latency. SWS seems to remain unaffected. Validity of these results, however, is diminished by methodological problems and the limited number of studies.

Atypical Antipsychotics

Quetiapine, which is approved for the treatment of schizophrenia, acute depressive, manic, and mixed episodes of bipolar I disorder, and as

Table 2
Antipsychotic classes and their sleep-related pharmacologic profiles

Medication/Class	Sleep-related Pharmacology	Effects on Sleep Architecture
Typical antipsychotics	Dopamine 2 receptor antagonism, H 1 antagonism, anticholinergic	Increased TST, improved sleep efficiency, decreased SOL, decreased WASO, unaffected SWS, increased REM latency
Atypical antipsychotics	Dopamine 2 receptor antagonism, 5-HT 2 antagonism, H 1 antagonism	Increased TST, increased sleep efficiency, decreased SOL, decreased WASO, increased SWS

Adapted from Barkoukis TR, Matheson JK, Ferber R, et al, editors. Therapy in sleep medicine. Philadelphia: Elsevier Saunders; 2012.

adjunct treatment of MDD, exhibits strong histamine (H1)-receptor antagonism and moderate affinity for 5-hydroxytryptamine (5-HT) serotonin type 2A receptors.[46] Antagonism at these sites is thought to be responsible for quetiapine's sedative effects.

In a meta-analysis of the numbers needed to treat to harm (NNTH) for discontinuation due to sedation,[47] both quetiapine-IR 300 mg per day and 600 mg per day resulted in significant risk of sedation with NNTH of 8 for both doses in patients with bipolar depression. NNTH with quetiapine-XR 150 mg per day and 300 mg per day in patients with refractory MDD were 9 and 7, respectively. NNTH with quetiapine-XR 50 mg per day, 150 mg per day, and 300 mg per day in patients with nonrefractory MDD were 5, 3, and 4, respectively.

In an open-label pilot study,[48] 18 adults with insomnia were treated with quetiapine 25 mg at bedtime, with dosages being increased to 50 mg in 7 patients and 75 mg in 1 patient. There were improvements in subjective and objective sleep parameters after 2 weeks that continued at 6 weeks. TST and sleep efficiency evaluated by polysomnography were significantly improved at 2 and 6 weeks. Pittsburgh Sleep Quality Index (PSQI) scores and subscores were also statistically improved at 2 and 6 weeks. Transient morning hangover was noted as a frequently reported adverse effect.

In non-PSG-based studies in patients with posttraumatic stress disorder, relatively low doses of quetiapine were associated with improvement in the PSQI global sleep score: sleep quality was subjectively better; SOL was reduced; TST improved; and episodes of terror and acting out dreams were reduced.[49]

In patients with schizophrenia, clozapine, which is sedating, has been noted to reduce SOL and increase TST and sleep efficiency.[50] In a population of treatment-refractory patients with bipolar disorder, the average time of going to bed was 55 minutes earlier with clozapine compared with that reported at baseline.[51] Similarly, risperidone has been shown to improve sleep maintenance and to decrease WASO in patients with schizophrenia.[52]

A 14-day PSG study evaluating the effects of paliperidone ER was conducted in a group of patients with schizophrenia-related insomnia.[53] In this double-blind, randomized, placebo-controlled study, paliperidone ER resulted in clinically and statistically significant differences in sleep measurements from baseline. There were significant reductions in SOL, WASO, time awake in bed, and stage 1 sleep duration. In addition, there was a prolongation of TST, stage 2 sleep duration, and REM sleep duration, and an increase in sleep efficiency index. Compared with placebo, paliperidone ER did not exacerbate daytime somnolence. Overall, it was well tolerated and improved sleep architecture and sleep continuity in this group of patients with schizophrenia and concomitant insomnia.

PSG studies in patients treated with olanzapine have shown significant decreases in wake time and stage 1 sleep and significant increases in TST, stage 2 sleep, and SWS (**Fig. 5**).[54,55]

RESTLESS LEGS SYNDROME

Antipsychotic agents may cause or exacerbate RLS.[50] A case series of 7 patients given low-dose quetiapine reported a dose-dependent provocation of RLS.[56] The investigators noted that most of these patients suffered from affective disorders and were on concomitant antidepressants. The Prescribing Information for quetiapine notes the occurrence of restless legs syndrome (RLS) in 2% of persons on quetiapine versus none on placebo.[57] Other case reports also seem to suggest that patients with affective disorders who are taking antidepressants may be particularly susceptible to the development of RLS.

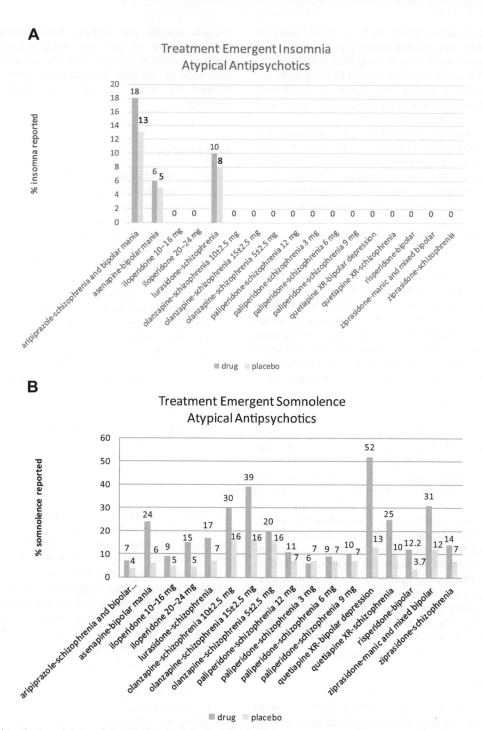

Fig. 5. (*A, B*) Complaints of treatment emergent somnolence are common with most antipsychotics. Caution should be taken in using these figures to predict the incidence of adverse effects in usual clinical practice where conditions and patient characteristics may differ from those in the respective clinical trials. In addition, results are not strictly comparative because they are derived from separate studies performed under differing conditions and with different methodologies. (*Data from* US Food and Drug Administration. FDA Approved Drug Products. Available at: http://www.accessdata.fda.gov/scripts/cder/drugsatfda/index.cfm. Accessed October 2, 2015.)

Antidepressant-induced RLS is most likely to occur with mirtazapine, which can be associated with provoking or deteriorating RLS in 28% of patients.[58] Antidepressant-induced RLS typically occurs within the first few days of treatment. Antidepressants are more likely to be associated with RLS in men than in women.[59]

It has been suggested that RLS is related to the dopaminergic effects of antidepressants.[60] These investigators suggested sertraline may be least likely among the SSRIs to cause RLS because it blocks dopamine reuptake. Bupropion may reduce RLS by increasing dopaminergic activity.[61]

NONBENZODIAZEPINE HYPNOTICS

Parasomnias like sleepwalking and sleep-related eating disorders (SRED) have been reported with nonbenzodiazepine hypnotics. In a review of parasomnias in psychiatric outpatients,[62] sleepwalking was linked to zolpidem and zopiclone, whereas both sleepwalking and SRED were associated with zolpidem alone. Parasomnias with this class of medication were more likely in patients taking them regularly rather than on an as-needed basis.

STIMULANTS

Stimulants are commonly prescribed for the treatment of attention-deficit/hyperactivity disorder (ADHD). The relationship between sleep and medication in children with ADHD is complex. Insomnia or delayed SOL greater than 30 minutes is one of the most common adverse effects associated with stimulant medications.[63] However, the effects of methylphenidate on sleep may depend on the length of time the child has been on the medication.[64] In addition, there are reports of children having difficulty falling asleep when the medication is being weaned off as well as children who fall asleep easily after taking a low dose of medication.[65] Results of polysomnographic studies in children with ADHD who were receiving methylphenidate have been inconsistent.[66]

SUMMARY

Antidepressant and antipsychotic agents frequently result in sleep-related adverse effects, primarily insomnia and daytime somnolence. However, these effects have not been well evaluated. Data from placebo-controlled trials are available primarily in the form of spontaneous reports rather than systematic assessments. Where sleep-related effects have been specifically studied as end points, the data are limited to small sample sizes and with methodological inconsistencies. In addition, comparative data between various agents are lacking. Nevertheless, the data available do provide some guidance regarding possible adverse effects on sleep and wakefulness, so that a therapeutic plan can be crafted for each patient's individual clinical situation.

REFERENCES

1. Benca RM, Obermeyer WH, Thisted RA, et al. Sleep and psychiatric disorders. A meta-analysis. Arch Gen Psychiatry 1992;49(8):651–68.
2. Pratt LA, Brody DJ, Gu Q. Antidepressant Use in Persons Aged 12 and Over: United States, 2005–2008. Hyattsville (MD): U.S. Department of Health and Human Services; Centers for Disease Control and Prevention; 2011. Available at: http://www.cdc.gov/nchs/data/databriefs/db76.pdf.
3. Saper CB, Scammell TE, Lu J. Hypothalamic regulation of sleep and circadian rhythms. Nature 2005; 437(7063):1257–63.
4. Fuller PM, Gooley JJ, Saper CB. Neurobiology of the sleep-wake cycle: sleep architecture, circadian regulation, and regulatory feedback. J Biol Rhythms 2006;21(6):482–93.
5. Berry RB, Brooks R, Gamaldo CE, et al, for the American Academy of Sleep Medicine. The AASM manual for the scoring of sleep and associated events: rules, terminology and technical specifications, version 2.2. Darien (IL): American Academy of Sleep Medicine; 2015. Available at: www.aasmnet.org.
6. Beasley CM Jr, Sayler ME, Weiss AM, et al. Fluoxetine: activating and sedating effects at multiple fixed doses. J Clin Psychopharmacol 1992;12(5):328–33.
7. Armitage R, Rush AJ, Trivedi M, et al. The effects of nefazodone on sleep architecture in depression. Neuropsychopharmacology 1994;10(2):123–7.
8. Kerkhofs M, Rielaert C, De Maertelaer V, et al. Fluoxetine in major depression: efficacy, safety and effects on sleep polygraphic variables. Int Clin Psychopharmacol 1990;5:253–60.
9. Hendrickse WA, Roffwarg HP, Grannemann BD, et al. The effects of fluoxetine on the polysomnogram of depressed outpatients: a pilot study. Neuropsychopharmacology 1994;10(2):85–91.
10. Gillin JC, Rapaport M, Erman MK, et al. A comparison of nefazodone and fluoxetine on mood and on objective, subjective, and clinician-rated measures of sleep in depressed patients: a double-blind, 8-week clinical trial. J Clin Psychiatry 1997;58(5):185–92.
11. Trivedi MH, Rush AJ, Armitage R, et al. Effects of fluoxetine on the polysomnogram in outpatients with major depression. Neuropsychopharmacology 1999;20(5):447–59.

12. Keck PE Jr, Hudson JI, Dorsey CM, et al. Effect of fluoxetine on sleep. Biol Psychiatry 1991;29(6):618–9.

13. Schenck CH, Mahowald MW, Kim SW, et al. Prominent eye movements during NREM sleep and REM sleep behavior disorder associated with fluoxetine treatment of depression and obsessive-compulsive disorder. Sleep 1992;15(3):226–35.

14. Dorsey CM, Lukas SE, Cunningham SL. Fluoxetine-induced sleep disturbance in depressed patients. Neuropsychopharmacology 1996;14(6):437–42.

15. Vasar V, Appelberg B, Rimon R, et al. The effect of fluoxetine on sleep: a longitudinal, double-blind polysomnographic study of healthy volunteers. Int Clin Psychopharmacol 1994;9(3):203–6.

16. Luthringer R, Toussaint M, Schaltenbrand N, et al. A double-blind, placebo-controlled evaluation of the effects of orally administered venlafaxine on sleep in inpatients with major depression. Psychopharmacol Bull 1996;32(4):637–46.

17. Salin-Pascual RJ, Galicia-Polo L, Drucker-Colin R. Sleep changes after 4 consecutive days of venlafaxine administration in normal volunteers. J Clin Psychiatry 1997;58(8):348–50.

18. Mouret J, Lemoine P, Minuit MP, et al. Effects of trazodone on the sleep of depressed subjects–a polygraphic study. Psychopharmacology 1988;95(Suppl):S37–43.

19. Organon, Inc. Remeron—a novel pharmacological treatment for depression. West Orange (NJ): Organon, Inc; 1996.

20. Kent JM. SNaRIs, NaSSAs, and NaRIs: new agents for the treatment of depression. Lancet (London, England) 2000;355(9207):911–8.

21. Grasmader K, Verwohlt PL, Kuhn KU, et al. Relationship between mirtazapine dose, plasma concentration, response, and side effects in clinical practice. Pharmacopsychiatry 2005;38(3):113–7.

22. Winokur A, Sateia MJ, Hayes JB, et al. Acute effects of mirtazapine on sleep continuity and sleep architecture in depressed patients: a pilot study. Biol Psychiatry 2000;48(1):75–8.

23. Organon USA. Product information REMERON oral tablets, mirtazapine tablets. Roseland (NJ): Organon USA, Inc; 2007.

24. Nofzinger EA, Reynolds CF 3rd, Thase ME, et al. REM sleep enhancement by bupropion in depressed men. Am J Psychiatry 1995;152(2):274–6.

25. Forest Pharmaceuticals USA, Inc. Product information for FETZIMA (levomilnacipran) extended-release capsules. St Louis (MO): Forest Pharmaceuticals USA, Inc; 2013.

26. Forest Pharmaceuticals USA, Inc. Product information for VIIBRYD (vilazodone hydrochloride) tablets. Cincinnati (OH): Forest Pharmaceuticals USA, Inc; 2015.

27. Takeda Pharmaceuticals America, Inc. Product information for BRINTELLIX (vortioxetine) tablets. Deerfield (IL): Takeda Pharmaceuticals America, Inc; 2013.

28. Kupfer DJ, Spiker DG, Rossi A, et al. Nortriptyline and EEG sleep in depressed patients. Biol Psychiatry 1982;17(5):535–46.

29. Shipley JE, Kupfer DJ, Dealy RS, et al. Differential effects of amitriptyline and of zimelidine on the sleep electroencephalogram of depressed patients. Clin Pharmacol Ther 1984;36(2):251–9.

30. Ware JC, Brown FW, Moorad PJ Jr, et al. Effects on sleep: a double-blind study comparing trimipramine to imipramine in depressed insomniac patients. Sleep 1989;12(6):537–49.

31. Kupfer DJ, Perel JM, Pollock BG, et al. Fluvoxamine versus desipramine: Comparative polysomnographic effects. Biol Psychiatry 1991;29(1):23–40.

32. Markov D, Doghramji K. Doxepin for insomnia. Curr Psychiatry 2010;9(10):67–77.

33. Roth T, Rogowski R, Hull S, et al. Efficacy and safety of doxepin 1 mg, 3 mg, and 6 mg in adults with primary insomnia. Sleep 2007;30(11):1555–61.

34. Scharf M, Rogowski R, Hull S, et al. Efficacy and safety of doxepin 1 mg, 3 mg, and 6 mg in elderly patients with primary insomnia: a randomized, double-blind, placebo controlled crossover study. J Clin Psychiatry 2008;69:1557–64.

35. Vogel GW, Buffenstein A, Minter K, et al. Drug effects on REM sleep and on endogenous depression. Neurosci Biobehav Rev 1990;14(1):49–63.

36. Nofzinger EA, Schwartz RM, Reynolds CF 3rd, et al. Affect intensity and phasic REM sleep in depressed men before and after treatment with cognitive-behavioral therapy. J Consult Clin Psychol 1994;62(1):83–91.

37. Sharpley AL, Cowen PJ. Effect of pharmacologic treatments on the sleep of depressed patients. Biol Psychiatry 1995;37(2):85–98.

38. Reynolds CF 3rd, Buysse DJ, Brunner DP, et al. Maintenance nortriptyline effects on electroencephalographic sleep in elderly patients with recurrent major depression: double-blind, placebo- and plasma-level-controlled evaluation. Biol Psychiatry 1997;42(7):560–7.

39. Taylor MP, Reynolds CF 3rd, Frank E, et al. EEG sleep measures in later-life bereavement depression. A randomized, double-blind, placebo-controlled evaluation of nortriptyline. Am J Geriatr Psychiatry 1999;7(1):41–7.

40. Wyatt RJ, Fram DH, Kupfer DJ, et al. Total prolonged drug-induced REM sleep suppression in anxious-depressed patients. Arch Gen Psychiatry 1971;24(2):145–55.

41. Kupfer DJ, Bowers MB Jr. REM sleep and central monoamine oxidase inhibition. Psychopharmacologia 1972;27(3):183–90.

42. Monti JM. Effect of a reversible monoamine oxidase-A inhibitor (moclobemide) on sleep of depressed patients. Br J Psychiatry Suppl 1989;(6):61–5.

43. Wetter TC, Lauer CJ, Gillich G, et al. The electroencephalographic sleep pattern in schizophrenic patients treated with clozapine or classical antipsychotic drugs. J Psychiatr Res 1996;30(6):411–9.

44. Hinze-Selch D, Mullington J, Orth A, et al. Effects of clozapine on sleep: a longitudinal study. Biol Psychiatry 1997;42(4):260–6.

45. Touyz SW, Saayman GS, Zabow T. A psychophysiological investigation of the long-term effects of clozapine upon sleep patterns of normal young adults. Psychopharmacology 1978; 56(1):69–73.

46. Stahl SM. Selective histamine H1 antagonism: novel hypnotic and pharmacologic actions challenge classical notions of antihistamines. CNS Spectr 2008;13: 1027–38.

47. Gao K, Kemp DE, Fein E, et al. Number needed to treat to harm for discontinuation due to adverse events in the treatment of bipolar depression, major depressive disorder, and generalized anxiety disorder with atypical antipsychotics. J Clin Psychiatry 2011;72(8):1063–71.

48. Wiegand MH, Landry F, Bruckner T, et al. Quetiapine in primary insomnia: a pilot study. Psychopharmacology 2008;196(2):337–8.

49. Robert S, Hamner MB, Kose S, et al. Quetiapine improves sleep disturbances in combat veterans with PTSD: sleep data from a prospective, open-label study. J Clin Psychopharmacol 2005;25(4):387–8.

50. Krystal AD, Goforth HW, Roth T. Effects of antipsychotic medications on sleep in schizophrenia. Int Clin Psychopharmacol 2008;23(3):150–60.

51. Armitage R, Cole D, Suppes T, et al. Effects of clozapine on sleep in bipolar and schizoaffective disorders. Prog NeuroPsychopharmacol Biol Psychiatry 2004;28(7):1065–70.

52. Dursun SM, Patel JK, Burke JG, et al. Effects of typical antipsychotic drugs and risperidone on the quality of sleep in patients with schizophrenia: a pilot study. J Psychiatry Neurosci 1999;24(4):333–7.

53. Luthringer R, Staner L, Noel N, et al. A double-blind, placebo-controlled, randomized study evaluating the effect of paliperidone extended-release tablets on sleep architecture in patients with schizophrenia. Int Clin Psychopharmacol 2007;22(5):299–308.

54. Sharpley AL, Vassallo CM, Cowen PJ. Olanzapine increases slow-wave sleep: Evidence for blockade of central 5-HT(2C) receptors in vivo. Biol Psychiatry 2000;47(5):468–70.

55. Salin-Pascual RJ, Herrera-Estrella M, Galicia-Polo L, et al. Olanzapine acute administration in schizophrenic patients increases delta sleep and sleep efficiency. Biol Psychiatry 1999;46(1):141–3.

56. Rittmannsberger H, Werl R. Restless legs syndrome induced by quetiapine: report of seven cases and review of the literature. Int J Neuropsychopharmacol 2013;16:1427–31.

57. AstraZeneca Pharmaceuticals LP. Product information for SEROQUEL (quetiapine fumarate) tablets. Wilmington (DE): AstraZeneca Pharmaceuticals LP; 2009.

58. Rottach KG, Schaner BM, Kirch MH, et al. Restless legs syndrome as side effect of second generation antidepressants. J Psychiatr Res 2008;43(1):70–5.

59. Baughman KR, Bourguet CC, Ober SK. Gender differences in the association between antidepressant use and restless legs syndrome. Mov Disord 2009; 24(7):1054–9.

60. Perroud N, Lazignac C, Baleydier B, et al. Restless legs syndrome induced by citalopram: a psychiatric emergency? Gen Hosp Psychiatry 2007;29(1):72–4.

61. Kim SW, Shin IS, Kim JM, et al. Bupropion may improve restless legs syndrome: a report of three cases. Clin Neuropharmacol 2005;28(6):298–301.

62. Lam SP, Fong SY, Ho CK, et al. Parasomnia among psychiatric outpatients: a clinical, epidemiologic, cross-sectional study. J Clin Psychiatry 2008;69(9): 1374–82.

63. Stein MA. Unravelling sleep problems in treated and untreated children with ADHD. J Child Adolesc Psychopharmacol 1999;9(3):157–68.

64. Wigal SB, Wong AA, Jun A, et al. Adverse events in medication treatment-naive children with attention-deficit/hyperactivity disorder: results from a small, controlled trial of lisdexamfetamine dimesylate. J Child Adolesc Psychopharmacol 2012;22(2):149–56.

65. Chatoor I, Wells KC, Conners CK, et al. The effects of nocturnally administered stimulant medication on EEG sleep and behavior in hyperactive children. J Am Acad Child Psychiatry 1983;22(4):337–42.

66. Sadeh A, Pergamin L, Bar-Haim Y. Sleep in children with attention-deficit hyperactivity disorder: a meta-analysis of polysomnographic studies. Sleep Med Rev 2006;10(6):381–98.

Development of a Behavioral Sleep Intervention as a Novel Approach for Pediatric Obesity in School-aged Children

Chantelle N. Hart, PhD[a],*, Nicola L. Hawley, PhD[b],
Rena R. Wing, PhD[c]

KEYWORDS

- Obesity • Pediatrics • Sleep • Behavioral intervention

KEY POINTS

- Use of multiple methodological approaches for determining the potential efficacy of a novel approach for pediatric obesity prevention and treatment can provide a strong foundation and rationale for refining approaches and current treatment targets.
- Systematic study of how sleep duration may affect eating and activity pathways suggests that sleep may be an important modifiable risk factor for obesity prevention and treatment.
- Several future directions are warranted, including further refinement of behavioral interventions, and further delineation of the mechanisms through which sleep may affect obesity risk.

INTRODUCTION

Despite being the focus of widespread public health efforts, childhood obesity remains an epidemic worldwide. The most recent US estimates show that 17.7% (95% confidence interval [CI], 14.5–21.4) of children 6 to 11 years old are obese (body mass index for age ≥95th Centers for Disease Control and Prevention [CDC] percentile), whereas a further 16.5% are overweight and at risk for becoming obese.[1] Given the now well-documented consequences of obesity for childhood health and psychosocial functioning, as well

as associated morbidity in adulthood, identifying novel, modifiable behaviors that can be targeted to improve weight control is imperative.

The observation that while obesity levels were increasing, the duration of children's nighttime sleep was decreasing,[2] accompanied by compelling evidence for the potential role of sleep in both intake and expenditure aspects of energy balance,[3–7] suggests that nighttime sleep might be one such modifiable factor. Numerous cross-sectional and prospective observational studies have supported the association between sleep duration and obesity risk in children.[8–10] A recent

This article originally appeared in *Pediatric Clinics of North America*, Volume 63, Issue 3, June 2016.
Disclosures: None.
[a] Department of Social and Behavioral Sciences, Center for Obesity Research and Education, College of Public Health, Temple University, 3223 North Broad Street, Philadelphia, PA 19140, USA; [b] Department of Chronic Disease Epidemiology, Yale School of Public Health, 60 College Street, New Haven, CT 06520, USA; [c] Department of Psychiatry and Human Behavior, Weight Control and Diabetes Research Center, The Miriam Hospital, Alpert Medical School of Brown University, 196 Richmond Street, Providence, RI 02903, USA
* Corresponding author.
E-mail address: chantelle.hart@temple.edu

meta-analysis found that, across 22 prospective observational studies of children aged 6 months to 18 years at baseline, from diverse backgrounds, children with a shorter sleep duration had twice the risk of overweight/obesity (odds ratio [OR], 2.15; 95% CI, 1.64–2.81) compared with their longer-sleeping peers.[10] The association was stronger among younger (OR, 1.88; 95% CI, 1.26–2.81) compared with older children (OR, 1.55; 95% CI, 1.22–1.97).[10]

Several pathways have been suggested that may link short sleep with obesity risk,[11] (**Fig. 1**). Experimental studies in healthy adults have provided evidence that sleep restriction or deprivation results in several neuroendocrine and inflammatory changes: impaired glucose metabolism, reduced insulin sensitivity, and increased levels of inflammatory mediators such as interleukin-6 and tumor necrosis factor.[12–14] Of particular interest are the changes that occur in hormones related to hunger and appetite; sleep restriction has been shown to reduce levels of leptin, a hunger inhibitor, and increase levels of the hunger hormone ghrelin.[6,7,15–17] Additional pathways proposed, and supported at least in part by adult experimental studies, include poorer food choices among those who are sleep deprived as well as reduced activity levels related to daytime tiredness.[3–7] Pediatric observational studies[18–23] are consistent with adult experimental studies, suggesting that similar pathways may be responsible for associations between short sleep and obesity risk in children as well. However, the pediatric literature remains limited by the observational nature of most of the existing studies.

To build on previous work, our group developed Project SLEEP, a series of studies designed to determine whether changes in children's sleep lead to changes in eating and activity habits and weight status. The approach was grounded in behavioral theory and informed by empirically supported treatment approaches for pediatric sleep disorders.[24–28] Importantly, studies were designed to systematically build on each other, and to test hypotheses using 2 distinct approaches: (1) an experimental research design, and (2) randomized controlled trials to evaluate relative efficacy of behavioral interventions. The experimental study[29] enabled careful manipulation of children's sleep to create large discrepancies in sleep duration and thus optimize detection of the impact of sleep on eating pathways associated with obesity risk. Given the need for translation of epidemiologic findings for development of a novel approach for prevention and/or treatment of pediatric obesity, randomized controlled trials allowed for piloting of a novel behavioral intervention to enhance sleep. Findings from these studies, the process undertaken to move from one study to the next, and future directions for this work are discussed below.

Commonalities Across Studies

The studies described below were designed with an eye toward dissemination. As such, to enhance ecological validity, all studies were conducted with children sleeping at home and coming into the research center for assessment and intervention visits only. Further, all studies enrolled both children who were normal weight and overweight/obese given that epidemiologic studies have shown that long sleep is protective against subsequent change in weight status in both normal-weight and overweight/obese children.[30,31] Thus inclusion of children drawn from both populations increased the ability to generalize findings for both prevention and treatment of obesity.

In addition, all studies enrolled children who reported sleeping approximately 9.5 h/night (or less).

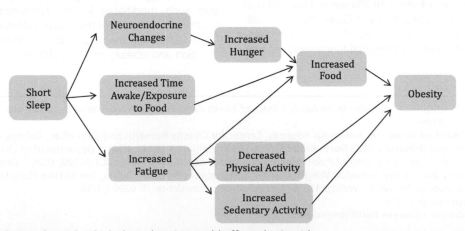

Fig. 1. Pathways through which sleep duration could affect obesity risk.

This criterion was used because children in the United States report sleeping approximately 9.5 h/night on average,[32,33] which is less than what has been recommended (ie, 10–11 h/night)[34,35] for children 8 to 11 years old, which is the population of interest in these studies. Thus, as with the decision regarding enrollment by weight status, establishing a criterion for sleep at 9.5 h/night enabled greater ability to generalize findings. Importantly, in the experimental study, enrolling children who slept approximately 9.5 h/night allowed for both sleep extension and restriction by 1.5 h/night without reaching a ceiling for how much sleep children this age could achieve while also not sleep depriving them too much. In terms of the behavioral interventions, enrolling children who slept 9.5 hours or less allowed sufficient room to potentially enhance sleep using behavioral strategies.

In addition, across all studies the authors differentiated between 2 sleep constructs: time in bed (TIB) and the actigraph sleep period. Because children cannot be forced to sleep, but it is possible to prescribe when they should be in bed with the lights out and attempting to sleep, all prescriptions for changes in sleep were made by changing children's TIB (ie, the time between their lights being turned off and the child trying to fall asleep and waking the next morning). However, the primary outcome of interest across all studies was change in the objective assessment of sleep: the actigraph sleep period (ie, the time between when the actigraph estimates sleep onset and offset).

Study 1 Development: Can Sleep Be Enhanced in Otherwise Healthy Children?

Several studies, primarily with preschool children, show that brief behavioral interventions can promote healthier sleep in children diagnosed with behavioral sleep disorders.[25,26,36–39] However, there is limited evidence for the efficacy of behavioral intervention to enhance sleep in otherwise healthy school-aged children who are reported to have insufficient sleep. Thus the goal of study 1 was to determine whether a brief behavioral intervention could enhance sleep in short-sleeping children. Given that it was a first evaluation of the newly designed intervention (described later; Table 1) it focused on acute changes in sleep. With an eye toward obesity prevention/treatment, it also focused on whether changes in sleep affected children's eating behaviors. We assessed the relative reinforcing value (RRV) of food, which provided an objective measure of motivation for an energy-dense food reward.

Fourteen children 8 to 11 years old who slept 9.5 h/night or less most nights of the week were enrolled into this 3-week pilot study. Following a 1-week baseline assessment, children were randomized to either increase their TIB by 1.5 h/night or continue with their current sleep habits. The 1.5-hour TIB increase was a prescription designed to maximize children's ability to achieve an increase in the actigraph sleep period of at least 45 min/night (ie, estimating sleep onset latency of 20–25 minutes and not expecting children to have perfect adherence to the prescribed change in TIB). Intervention families were provided with effective behavioral strategies to increase TIB, and returned after 1 week to assess adherence and problem-solve regarding barriers. Table 1 details the effective behavioral strategies used in this study. A 2:1 (intervention/control) randomization scheme was used to ensure adequate samples to assess intervention efficacy. All children returned again 2 weeks after baseline for the follow-up assessment. Primary variables of interest were change in the actigraph sleep period and change in food reinforcement (ie, how motivated a child was for a food reward). The Behavioral Choice Task,[40] a validated computer-based measure, was used to assess food reinforcement.[41–43] In this pilot, we were specifically interested in the RRV of energy-dense snack foods compared with sedentary activities (that were equally liked).

Twelve (86%) children had complete study data (1 child did not attend the 2-week assessment, and an actigraph malfunctioned in a second child). Children were 9.2 ± 1.1 years old with a mean body mass index (BMI) percentile (using CDC norms) of 71.7 ± 29.3 (58% overweight/obese); 75% were male, and 66% were non-Hispanic white. As shown in Fig. 2, children in the intervention condition increased their actigraph sleep period by 40 ± 22 min/night versus a decrease (−16 ± 30 min/night) in control participants (t = 3.77; P = .004; d = 2.30). Children in the intervention tended to decrease the proportion of points earned for a food reward (−0.09 ± 0.21), whereas children in the control group showed no change (0.006 ± 0.04; t = −1.09; nonsignificant; d = 0.56) (Fig. 3). Although this change in the RRV of food was not significant, it represents a medium-sized effect.

In summary, this study showed that our intervention was able to acutely enhance school-aged children's sleep. Importantly, there were no observed or reported negative effects of intervention, such as longer sleep onset latency or greater percentage of time lying awake in bed. Further, there was also a signal that changes in sleep could lead to changes in children's motivation for food.

Table 1
Behavioral intervention components employed in studies 1 and 3

Behavioral Strategy	Operationalization
Goal setting	Families are prescribed a 1–1.5 h increase in children's TIB, which is based on family reported TIB achieved at baseline and confirmed with actigraphy
Preplanning	Although the behavioral goal for TIB is prescriptive, interventionists preplan with families how best to achieve the goal given schedules and life circumstances. Flexibility is afforded on weekends (ie, children are allowed to stay up 1 h later as long as they can sleep in the next day for an additional hour)
Self-monitoring	Families are provided with sleep diaries in which they document the time lights are turned off and the child is trying to fall asleep, time the child wakes up, and time the child gets out of bed. Monitoring of mood, aberrations during the day (eg, vacation day from school, illness), and activities included in bedtime routines is also included
Problem solving	Both facilitators and barriers to achieving the behavioral goals are identified. Intervention staff work with families to help them identify strategies for maximizing facilitators and minimizing likelihood of barriers to behavior change
Positive reinforcement	Positive reinforcement is woven throughout the intervention. Intervention staff positively reinforce families throughout intervention sessions, parents are taught to do the same at home throughout the duration of the study, and a sticker chart with family-focused, nonmonetary (or minimally priced) rewards is used to encourage children to make changes in their TIB
Positive routine	To promote sleep onset, families are encouraged to develop a bedtime routine of approximately 20–30 min that includes the use of a routine set of behaviors that can serve as cues for sleep onset (eg, brushing teeth, getting pajamas on, reading a book together)
Sleep hygiene/stimulus control strategies	In addition to positive routines, several stimulus control strategies are reviewed and recommended to enhance the likelihood of adherence to the prescribed changes in TIB. These strategies include a consistent sleep schedule, no caffeine within at least 2 h of bedtime, no screen time as part of the bedtime routine, removing televisions and other light-emitting devices from bedrooms, and using beds only for sleeping (eg, no homework in bed)

Thus these encouraging results suggested the need to continue to evaluate the potential utility of sleep in enhancing children's weight-related behaviors. However, findings were limited by the focus on acute (2-week) changes in sleep in a small sample of children. Further, it was challenging reviewing with families all of the behavioral strategies (eg, goal setting, stimulus control/sleep

hygiene, self-monitoring, and positive reinforcement) in a single visit of 45 to 60 minutes. Thus, to enhance potential efficacy, the intervention needed to be refined to deliver the behavioral

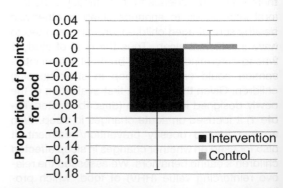

Fig. 2. Mean between-groups change in actigraph sleep period. F/U, follow-up.

Fig. 3. Mean between-groups change in the RRV of food.

content across greater than 1 treatment session. Further, to strengthen rationale it would be important to show that changes in sleep could be maintained over longer periods of time and with a larger sample of children. In addition, although the primary focus of study 1 was to determine whether sleep could be enhanced in otherwise healthy children, it was not designed to create large changes in sleep to maximize the ability to detect whether changes in sleep affect changes in several potential pathways through which sleep may affect obesity risk.

Study 2 Preliminary Testing: Experimental Changes in Sleep, Eating, and Weight

As study 1 was closing, study 2, which used an experimental design, was being launched. As noted earlier, this second study, a proof-of-concept study, was designed to maximize differences in children's sleep to allow detection of how sleep may affect obesity risk, primarily through eating pathways. Primary findings have been previously reported; readers are referred to the main article for details.[29] In brief, 39 children were enrolled into a 3-week study. During the first week, children were asked to sleep their typical amount. This week served 2 main purposes: to ensure final eligibility for the study based on reported sleep length (confirmed with actigraphy), and to establish a starting point from which to prescribe changes in TIB during the experimental weeks. After the baseline week, children were randomized to either increase or decrease TIB by 1.5 h/night (thus, the goal was to create a 3-hour TIB difference between experimental conditions). All changes in TIB were made by changing bedtimes; wake times remained constant across all study weeks. In order to achieve high levels of participant adherence, several strategies were used, including prescription of bedtimes and wake times (which were closely monitored by study staff through a twice-daily call-in system) as well as children being paid to adhere to the sleep schedule.[29] Primary outcomes of interest were reported dietary intake (measured by 3-day 24-hour dietary recalls), fasting levels of leptin and ghrelin, and food reinforcement.

Thirty-seven of the 39 enrolled children completed the study. Findings showed high levels of adherence to the prescribed sleep schedule with a 141-minute difference in the actigraph sleep period between conditions.[29] Importantly, when children decreased their sleep, they reported consuming 134 kcal/d more (based on 3 days of 24-hour dietary recalls) and weighed approximately 0.22 kg (0.5 lb) more at the end of the

decreased week compared with their weight at the end of the increased week.[29] Most of the additional caloric intake was reportedly consumed during the additional hours awake in the evening during the decreased sleep condition. Despite these changes in reported caloric intake and measured weight, there were no differences in food reinforcement or in fasting ghrelin levels. Further, findings regarding leptin were contrary to hypotheses, which may have been caused by several factors, including energy balance not being maintained (ie, children's weight changed) and potential effects of the circadian timing system (given large shifts in bedtimes).[29]

Nonetheless, findings from this experimental study were encouraging. High levels of adherence to the prescribed changes in TIB and objective measures of sleep time allowed a valid comparison of how changes in sleep could affect changes in the study outcomes. Findings also provided a second signal that changes in sleep could affect changes in eating behaviors. Importantly, they also suggested that large changes in sleep could affect children's weight status. However, limitations were observed, including the focus, again, on acute changes in sleep duration and a small study sample as well as a lack of a wash-out period between experimental conditions. To determine clinical significance of preliminary findings, a larger trial that assesses how prescribed changes in TIB affect children's sleep, eating and activity behaviors, and weight status was needed.

Study 3 Efficacy: Does a Brief Behavioral Intervention Lead to Short-term Changes in Sleep, Eating and Activity Behaviors, and Weight Status?

To address limitations of the 2 previous studies, study 3, which is an ongoing, fully powered randomized controlled trial, was launched. Primary aims are to determine whether a brief behavioral intervention to increase sleep in school-aged children results in changes in the actigraph sleep period relative to control over a 2-month interval, and to determine the effect of intervention on eating and activity behaviors, and weight status. Specifically, we hypothesize that children randomized to the optimized sleep condition will show greater increases in the actigraph sleep period at 2 months than children in the control group. Second, children in the optimized sleep group will show a greater decrease in total caloric intake and percentage of their calories consumed as fat relative to controls. Additional secondary hypotheses are that the optimized sleep group will engage in more moderate-vigorous physical activity and less sedentary activity, that they will show a greater decrease in the RRV of food, and that they will show a greater decrease in BMI z-score compared with children in the control group.

One-hundred and four children aged 8 to 11 years who are reported by parents to sleep approximately 9.5 hours or less each night are being enrolled in the 2-month study. After completing a baseline assessment week during which eligibility based on reported TIB is confirmed with actigraphy, children are randomized in a 1:1 fashion to either the active behavioral intervention or a control for contact condition (ie, same number of visits as the intervention arm, but no discussion of enhancing sleep; just a focus on accurate completion of assessments and study procedures). As in study 1, children randomized to the intervention group are being asked to increase TIB by 1.5 h/night over the study period, and children in the control group are being asked to continue with current sleep behaviors. To extend findings from the first 2 studies, assessments are occurring at baseline, 2 weeks, and 2 months. At each assessment, sleep duration is being estimated using standard procedures for wrist-worn actigraphy to establish the actigraph sleep period[44,45]; dietary intake is being assessed with 3 days of 24-hour dietary recalls (using multiple pass methodology), and physical activity is being assessed with hip-worn accelerometry. Height and weight are being assessed by study staff using standard procedures and with children in light clothing and without shoes. In addition, food reinforcement is being assessed as in studies 1 and 2 with the Behavioral Choice task. Importantly, given findings from study 2 suggesting that changes in food intake were observed later in the day, assessments were moved from the morning to the late afternoon/early evening in an effort to capture potential changes in eating behaviors that may result from changes in sleep.

The sleep intervention mirrors the one developed and tested in study 1, but is being delivered across 4 sessions. Given the evidence from the prior studies and the wider sleep literature that a brief behavioral intervention can produce large changes in sleep,[25,26,36–39] 2 in-person intervention sessions are being provided (60 minutes and 30 minutes, respectively) delivered by a trained behavioral interventionist in the first 2 weeks postrandomization: the first immediately following randomization and the second 1 week later. Given findings from behavioral weight control interventions that early success predicts overall success in behavioral programs, this was done intentionally to support rapid changes in TIB. As in study 1, effective behavioral strategies were used to promote changes in TIB (see **Table 1**). In-person sessions are followed by phone follow-ups at 4 and 6 weeks postrandomization. These sessions focus primarily on reinforcing progress toward sleep goals, identifying facilitators and barriers to enhancing TIB, and problem solving to maximize facilitators and minimize risk of continued barriers.

Findings from this ongoing trial will provide important information regarding the efficacy of a brief behavioral intervention to produce sustainable changes in sleep over a 2-month period. By focusing on additional outcomes such as children's eating and activity behaviors and weight status, it will also allow assessment of whether enhancing children's sleep could have important implications for prevention and treatment of pediatric obesity.

SUMMARY/DISCUSSION

In summary, findings from the studies described earlier show that enhancing children's sleep may show promise in assisting with weight regulation. These findings are particularly encouraging given that different methodological approaches have been/are being used and that each study has built systematically on prior work. Although encouraging, several avenues of future study are warranted, including better delineation of the mechanisms through which sleep duration influences weight status, continued refinement of intervention targets, and evaluation of intervention efficacy over longer periods of time. Determination of the relative efficacy of sleep as an adjunct treatment approach for pediatric obesity may also be warranted.

Although several pathways through which sleep may affect obesity risk have been proposed, it will be important to more clearly specify potential mechanisms underlying this relationship. Doing so may not only help to strengthen the rationale for enhancing sleep as a means of affecting children's weight status, it may also help identify ways to further enhance intervention efficacy. For example, findings from our experimental study suggest that the additional hours awake may, at least in part, account for additional caloric intake when children's sleep is restricted.[29] This finding is consistent with other emerging work with adolescents[46] and adults,[3] and may suggest that the increased exposure to food-rich environments is a primary pathway through which short sleep affects obesity risk. As such, interventions focused on stimulus control efforts to minimize less healthy food options and potentially decrease the variety of foods available in the home may be an important adjunct treatment target. Alternatively, given large shifts that were made in children's bedtimes in study 2, the circadian timing system may also be influencing eating behaviors. Emerging work shows a potentially important role of the circadian system in eating behaviors, hormonal release and metabolism, and weight regulation.[47–49] Thus it is possible that shifts in circadian timing could affect study outcomes.

In addition to previously identified mechanisms, other unique mechanisms could account for how changes in sleep affect obesity risk. For example, one mechanism that has been associated with both sleep and obesity risk is executive functions (EF). It is notable that the association between sleep and obesity risk is strongest during a period of rapid growth in EF.[50,51] This observation is underscored by several studies that have shown independent associations between EF and both sleep[52,53] and obesity risk.[54,55] It has been suggested that sleep deprivation may lead to unhealthy eating behaviors and weight gain via changes in EF secondary to functional changes in the prefrontal cortex (PFC), specifically regions involved in reward and regulation of emotion and behavior. Imaging studies with adults support this hypothesis. When presented with food images, participants show, for example, increased activation in the right anterior cingulate cortex[56] and orbitofrontal cortex[57] when sleep is restricted (compared with a rested condition). These regions are involved in motivation, reinforcement, decision making, and self-control.[57] An additional study showed decreased activation to food images in the ventromedial PFC in individuals who reported greater daytime sleepiness (compared with those who were less sleepy), suggesting possible decreases in inhibition related to energy-dense foods when fatigued.[58] Thus insufficient sleep may predispose individuals to excessive caloric intake because the rewarding properties of food (particularly highly palatable foods)[17] strengthen; the ability to inhibit responses to energy-dense foods is impaired; and the ability to sustain goal-directed, healthy eating behaviors is compromised. This hypothesis is consistent with behavioral findings. Experimental studies with adults suggest that increased caloric intake is not caused by greater homeostatic need for energy, but by hedonic processes (ie, greater appetitive drive).[3,59,60] Enhancing sleep could therefore decrease excessive energy intake by decreasing the rewarding properties of food (an effect found in study 1), and enhancing individuals' ability to resist food temptations within the context of our food-rich environment. At present these potential pathways are speculative. It will be important to conduct additional studies to more definitively delineate underlying processes that may be at work.

Beyond the importance of identifying mechanisms, future work could continue to extend the present findings in several ways. Although study 3 is ongoing, if findings are consistent with previous studies, demonstration of persistence of treatment effects over longer periods of time will be important. This finding will be particularly relevant given that enhancing children's sleep for longer periods of time will likely be necessary to observe significant effects on weight-related outcomes. Given the need for translation of empirical findings to community settings, it will also be important to identify active treatment components. As noted earlier, our studies in this area affect both the duration of sleep and parameters that may optimize circadian functioning (ie, advancing bedtimes, promoting consistent sleep schedules). Thus it will be important to determine which component is driving the observed findings (or whether both are key) so that targeted messages can be developed to efficiently promote necessary behavior change. Given that this work has focused singularly on enhancing sleep duration, to maximize impact on weight outcomes, it will also be important to consider combining a brief behavioral sleep intervention with other established approaches and/or strategies for weight regulation (ie, as adjunct to standard behavioral weight control treatment and/or with targeted obesogenic behaviors). Such an approach may be key to understanding the utility of sleep at enhancing weight regulation, and maximizing the efficacy of brief approaches with high translation potential.

In conclusion, our developmental work related to the effect of enhancing sleep on weight-related outcomes suggests that sleep may play an important role in children's weight regulation. Although additional work is needed to more definitively identify sleep as a key behavior to enhance in an effort to decrease pediatric obesity risk, these preliminary studies, along with emerging work with adolescents and adults, provide a strong foundation for continued exploration.

ACKNOWLEDGMENTS

The authors acknowledge all of the collaborators involved in these studies, including Mary Carskadon, PhD; Hollie Raynor, PhD; Elissa Jelalian, PhD; Judith Owens, MD, MPH; Robert Considine, PhD; Joseph Fava, PhD; and Adam Davey, PhD. In addition, we thank the postdoctoral fellows and staff who ensured the success of each study, including Alyssa Cairns, PhD; Elizabeth Kuhl, PhD; Kathrin Osterholt Fedosov, MA; Brittany James; Jessica Lawton; Amanda Samuels; Victoria Mathieu; Zeely Denmat; Isabella Cassell; Risha

Kheterpal; Ashley Greer; Heather Polonsky; and Andrew Pool. We are also indebted to all of the participating families in these studies, without whom reporting of these findings would not be possible.

REFERENCES

1. Ogden CL, Carroll MD, Kit BK, et al. Prevalence of childhood and adult obesity in the United States, 2011-2012. JAMA 2014;311(8):806–14.
2. Matricciani L, Olds T, Petkov J. In search of lost sleep: secular trends in the sleep time of school-aged children and adolescents. Sleep Med Rev 2012;16(3):203–11.
3. Markwald RR, Melanson EL, Smith MR, et al. Impact of insufficient sleep on total daily energy expenditure, food intake, and weight gain. Proceedings of the National Academy of Sciences of the United States of America 2013;110(14):5695–700.
4. Brondel L, Romer MA, Nougues PM, et al. Acute partial sleep deprivation increases food intake in healthy men. Am J Clin Nutr 2010;91(6):1550–9.
5. St-Onge MP, Roberts AL, Chen J, et al. Short sleep duration increases energy intakes but does not change energy expenditure in normal-weight individuals. Am J Clin Nutr 2011;94(2):410–6.
6. Schmid SM, Hallschmid M, Jauch-Chara K, et al. A single night of sleep deprivation increases ghrelin levels and feelings of hunger in normal-weight healthy men. J Sleep Res 2008;17(3):331–4.
7. Benedict C, Hallschmid M, Lassen A, et al. Acute sleep deprivation reduces energy expenditure in healthy men. Am J Clin Nutr 2011;93(6):1229–36.
8. Cappuccio FP, Taggart FM, Kandala NB, et al. Meta-analysis of short sleep duration and obesity in children and adults. Sleep 2008;31(5):619–26.
9. Hart CN, Cairns A, Jelalian E. Sleep and obesity in children and adolescents. Pediatr Clin North Am 2011;58(3):715–33.
10. Fatima Y, Doi SA, Mamun AA. Longitudinal impact of sleep on overweight and obesity in children and adolescents: a systematic review and bias-adjusted meta-analysis. Obes Rev 2015;16(2):137–49.
11. Patel SR, Hu FB. Short sleep duration and weight gain: a systematic review. Obesity (Silver Spring) 2008;16(3):643–53.
12. Grandner MA, Sands-Lincoln MR, Pak VM, et al. Sleep duration, cardiovascular disease, and proinflammatory biomarkers. Nat Sci Sleep 2013;5: 93–107.
13. Nedeltcheva AV, Kessler L, Imperial J, et al. Exposure to recurrent sleep restriction in the setting of high caloric intake and physical inactivity results in increased insulin resistance and reduced glucose tolerance. J Clin Endocrinol Metab 2009;94(9): 3242–50.
14. Morselli LL, Guyon A, Spiegel K. Sleep and metabolic function. Pflügers Arch 2012;463(1):139–60.
15. Mullington JM, Haack M, Toth M, et al. Cardiovascular, inflammatory, and metabolic consequences of sleep deprivation. Prog Cardiovasc Dis 2009;51(4): 294–302.
16. Spiegel K, Leproult R, L'Hermite-Baleriaux M, et al. Leptin levels are dependent on sleep duration: relationships with sympathovagal balance, carbohydrate regulation, cortisol, and thyrotropin. J Clin Endocrinol Metab 2004;89(11):5762–71.
17. Spiegel K, Tasali E, Penev P, et al. Brief communication: sleep curtailment in healthy young men is associated with decreased leptin levels, elevated ghrelin levels, and increased hunger and appetite. Ann Intern Med 2004;141(11):846–50.
18. Androutsos O, Moschonis G, Mavrogianni C, et al. Identification of lifestyle patterns, including sleep deprivation, associated with insulin resistance in children: the Healthy Growth Study. Eur J Clin Nutr 2014;68(3):344–9.
19. Verhulst SL, Schrauwen N, Haentjens D, et al. Sleep duration and metabolic dysregulation in overweight children and adolescents. Arch Dis Child 2008; 93(1):89–90.
20. Javaheri S, Storfer-Isser A, Rosen CL, et al. Association of short and long sleep durations with insulin sensitivity in adolescents. J Pediatr 2011;158(4): 617–23.
21. Matthews KA, Dahl RE, Owens JF, et al. Sleep duration and insulin resistance in healthy black and white adolescents. Sleep 2012;35(10):1353–8.
22. Iglayreger HB, Peterson MD, Liu D, et al. Sleep duration predicts cardiometabolic risk in obese adolescents. J Pediatr 2014;164(5):1085–90.e1.
23. Leproult R, Van Cauter E. Role of sleep and sleep loss in hormonal release and metabolism. Endocr Dev 2010;17:11–21.
24. Burke RV, Kuhn BR, Peterson JL. Brief report: a "storybook" ending to children's bedtime problems–the use of a rewarding social story to reduce bedtime resistance and frequent night waking. J Pediatr Psychol 2004;29(5):389–96.
25. Kuhn BR, Elliott AJ. Treatment efficacy in behavioral pediatric sleep medicine. J Psychosom Res 2003; 54(6):587–97.
26. Mindell JA, Kuhn B, Lewin DS, et al. Behavioral treatment of bedtime problems and night wakings in infants and young children. Sleep 2006;29(10): 1263–76.
27. Sadeh A. Cognitive-behavioral treatment for childhood sleep disorders. Clin Psychol Rev 2005; 25(5):612–28.
28. Mindell JA. Empirically supported treatments in pediatric psychology: bedtime refusal and night wakings in young children. J Pediatr Psychol 1999; 24(6):465–81.

29. Hart CN, Carskadon MA, Considine RV, et al. Changes in children's sleep duration on food intake, weight, and leptin. Pediatrics 2013;132(6):e1473–80.

30. Agras WS, Hammer LD, McNicholas F, et al. Risk factors for childhood overweight: a prospective study from birth to 9.5 years. J Pediatr 2004; 145(1):20–5.

31. Snell EK, Adam EK, Duncan GJ. Sleep and the body mass index and overweight status of children and adolescents. Child Dev 2007;78(1):309–23.

32. Foundation NS. Final report: 2004 Sleep in America poll. 2004. Available at: http://www.sleepfoundation.org/_content//hottopics/2004SleepPollFinalReport.pdf. Accessed March 5, 2006.

33. Spilsbury JC, Storfer-Isser A, Drotar D, et al. Sleep behavior in an urban US sample of school-aged children. Arch Pediatr Adolesc Med 2004;158(10): 988–94.

34. Mindell JA, Owens J. A clinical guide to pediatric sleep: diagnosis and management of sleep problems. Philadelphia: Lippincott Williams & Wilkins; 2003.

35. Ferber R. Solve your child's sleep problems: new, revised and expanded edition. New York: Fireside; 1996.

36. Friman PC, Hoff KE, Schnoes C, et al. The bedtime pass: an approach to bedtime crying and leaving the room. Arch Pediatr Adolesc Med 1999;153(10): 1027–9.

37. Glaze DG. Childhood insomnia: why Chris can't sleep. Pediatr Clin North Am 2004;51(1):33–50, vi.

38. Owens JA, Palermo TM, Rosen CL. Overview of current management of sleep disturbance in children: II–behavioral interventions. Curr Ther Res 2002;63: B38–52.

39. Stores G. Practitioner review: assessment and treatment of sleep disorders in children and adolescents. J Child Psychol Psychiatry 1996;37(8):907–25.

40. Epstein L. Behavioral choice task: for measuring absolute and relative reinforcing value and habituation of operant behavior [computer program]. Buffalo, New York: State University of New York at Buffalo; 2007.

41. Raynor HA, Epstein LH. The relative-reinforcing value of food under differing levels of food deprivation and restriction. Appetite 2003;40(1):15–24.

42. Epstein LH, Truesdale R, Wojcik A, et al. Effects of deprivation on hedonics and reinforcing value of food. Physiol Behav 2003;78(2):221–7.

43. Saelens BE, Epstein LH. Reinforcing value of food in obese and non-obese women. Appetite 1996;27(1): 41–50.

44. Acebo C, LeBourgeois MK. Actigraphy. Respir Care Clin North Am 2006;12(1):23–30, viii.

45. Sadeh A. Assessment of intervention for infant night waking: parental reports and activity-based home monitoring. J Consult Clin Psychol 1994;62(1):63–8.

46. Beebe DW, Zhou A, Rausch J, et al. The impact of early bedtimes on adolescent caloric intake varies by chronotype. J Adolesc Health 2015;57(1):120–2.

47. Reutrakul S, Van Cauter E. Interactions between sleep, circadian function, and glucose metabolism: implications for risk and severity of diabetes. Ann N Y Acad Sci 2014;1311:151–73.

48. Morris CJ, Yang JN, Scheer FA. The impact of the circadian timing system on cardiovascular and metabolic function. Prog Brain Res 2012;199: 337–58.

49. Nohara K, Yoo S-H, Chen ZJ. Manipulating the circadian and sleep cycles to protect against metabolic disease. Front Endocrinol 2015;6:35.

50. Best JR, Miller PH. A developmental perspective on executive function. Child Dev 2010;81(6):1641–60.

51. Anderson P. Assessment and development of executive function (EF) during childhood. Child Neuropsychol 2002;8(2):71–82.

52. Randazzo AC, Muehlbach MJ, Schweitzer PK, et al. Cognitive function following acute sleep restriction in children ages 10-14. Sleep 1998;21(8):861–8.

53. Fallone G, Acebo C, Seifer R, et al. Experimental restriction of sleep opportunity in children: effects on teacher ratings. Sleep 2005;28(12):1561–7.

54. Temple JL, Legierski CM, Giacomelli AM, et al. Overweight children find food more reinforcing and consume more energy than do nonoverweight children. Am J Clin Nutr 2008;87(5):1121–7.

55. Bonato DP, Boland FJ. Delay of gratification in obese children. Addict Behav 1983;8(1):71–4.

56. Benedict C, Brooks SJ, O'Daly OG, et al. Acute sleep deprivation enhances the brain's response to hedonic food stimuli: an fMRI study. J Clin Endocrinol Metab 2012;97(3):E443–7.

57. St-Onge MP, McReynolds A, Trivedi ZB, et al. Sleep restriction leads to increased activation of brain regions sensitive to food stimuli. Am J Clin Nutr 2012;95(4):818–24.

58. Killgore WD, Schwab ZJ, Weber M, et al. Daytime sleepiness affects prefrontal regulation of food intake. Neuroimage 2013;71:216–23.

59. Chaput JP. Sleep patterns, diet quality and energy balance. Physiol Behav 2014;134:86–91.

60. Chaput JP. Is sleeping more and working less a new way to control our appetite? Eur J Clin Nutr 2010; 64(9):1032–3.

Testosterone Deficiency and Sleep Apnea

Omar Burschtin, MD[a], Jing Wang, MD[b],*

KEYWORDS

- Obstructive sleep apnea • Testosterone deficiency • Sexual dysfunction
- Continuous positive airway pressure

KEY POINTS

- Obstructive sleep apnea (OSA) is associated with altered pituitary–gonadal function.
- Serum testosterone (T) has been shown to be lower in men with OSA.
- T supplementation may alter ventilatory responses and reduce sensitivity to hypercapnea.
- OSA may be a risk factor for erectile and sexual dysfunction in men.
- Treatment of OSA may help improve hypogonadism and sexual function.

INTRODUCTION

Obstructive sleep apnea (OSA) is a common condition among middle-aged men, affecting approximately 25% of men over the age of 40 (apnea hypopnea index [AHI] >5).[1] When looking at more subtle divisions of OSA severity, 18% of men in this age group still fall within the mild category, at AHI greater than 10, and 11% have at least moderate disease, with AHI greater than 15. This disorder is characterized by repetitive collapse of the airway during sleep, resulting in oxygen desaturation and sleep fragmentation. Observational studies have shown that OSA is a risk factor for cardiovascular morbidity, including hypertension, coronary heart disease, and stroke.[2–4] Sleep-disordered breathing has also been associated with altered pituitary–gonadal function. This article discusses the relationship between OSA and testosterone (T) deficiency.

Studies evaluating the relationship between T and sleep date back to the 1970s.[5–7] One of the earlier studies measured T and luteinizing hormone (LH) every 20 minutes for 24 hours in 9 pubertal boys and 3 sexually mature young men, and found that T levels fluctuated over the course of the day, with pubertal boys showing an increase in LH and T secretion during sleep. When the sleep–wake cycle was reversed, this pattern held true. However, this effect was not seen in sexually mature men. Another study evaluated T levels in men aged 22 to 32 years after night sleep and daytime sleep, and found an increase in T levels during any period of sleep and a decrease during waking hours, independent of circadian timing.[8] These studies suggest that LH-T augmentation during sleep is an important component of normal male physiology.

LOW TESTOSTERONE AND SLEEP APNEA: ROLES OF AGE, BODY MASS INDEX, AND SEVERITY OF SLEEP APNEA

Serum T has been shown to be lower in men with OSA.[9] Multiple studies describe a negative correlation between polysomnographic parameters—AHI, oxygen desaturation index (ODI), and nadir oxygen saturation - and testosterone levels.[10,11] A study by Luboshitzky and colleagues, measuring LH and T between 7 p.m. and 7 a.m. in obese men with OSA, obese men without OSA, and lean healthy men, found LH and T to be significantly lower in obese men with OSA compared with lean controls. Furthermore, both men with

This article originally appeared in *Urologic Clinics of North America*, Volume 43, Issue 2, May 2016.
[a] Mount Sinai School of Medicine, Division of Pulmonary, Critical Care and Sleep Medicine, 11 East 26th Street, 13th Floor, New York, NY 10010, USA; [b] NYU School of Medicine, Division of Pulmonary, Critical Care, and Sleep Medicine, 462 First Avenue Room 7N24, New York, NY 10016, USA
* Corresponding author.
E-mail address: jing.wang@nyumc.org

Sleep Med Clin 11 (2016) 525–529
http://dx.doi.org/10.1016/j.jsmc.2016.08.003

OSA and middle-aged controls had less pulsatile T release and reduced LH pulse amplitude, suggesting that, beyond the presence of OSA, obesity and age also play a role in androgen secretion.[12]

LOW TESTOSTERONE AND SLEEP APNEA: ROLE OF FATIGUE

Fatigue is a common reported symptom in OSA, even in the absence of daytime sleepiness.[13] Bercea and colleagues investigated the relationship between fatigue, OSA, and T levels in 2 groups consisting of OSA patients and age- and body mass index (BMI)-matched controls without OSA. In addition to lower serum testosterone, severe OSA patients also had more general fatigue, physical fatigue, mental fatigue, and reduced activity. In multivariate analyses, T level was the only independent predictor of physical fatigue and reduced activity in the OSA group. Of note, nadir oxygen saturation was not a significant predictor of fatigue. This study suggests that T deficiency in men with OSA has multiple health consequences, and fatigue may be an important factor affecting quality of life in this cohort.[14]

EFFECT OF TESTOSTERONE SUPPLEMENTATION ON OBSTRUCTIVE SLEEP APNEA

Untreated OSA has been considered a contraindication to T therapy, as it is believed that T replacement therapy (TRT) can worsen sleep apnea. Several studies have investigated the role of T administration in OSA. A case study by Cistulli and colleagues[15] reported that administration of high-dose T to a 13-year-old boy exacerbated OSA due to neuromuscular collapse of upper airway during sleep. Schneider and colleagues[16] found an increase in the number of apneas and hypopneas and a corresponding rise in AHI following androgen administration to hypogonadal males. These changes were noted without significant changes in upper airway dimensions or alterations in sleep stage distribution.

Matsumoto and colleagues[17] evaluated the effect of 6 weeks of biweekly 200 mg intramuscular T enanthate injections on hypoxic and hypercapnic ventilatory drive (ie, increase in ventilation induced by hypoxia or hypercapnea) in 5 hypogonadal men. Hypoxic ventilatory drive decreased significantly, while hypercapnic ventilatory drive did not. OSA developed in 1 subject and worsened in another. Both these patients showed a decrease in oxygen saturation, development of cardiac dysrhythmias during sleep, and an increase in hematocrit. On retrospective review of another group of

elderly hypogonadal men with 2-year follow-up, a significant increase in hematocrit was seen, with 24% of men developing polycythemia (hematocrit [Hct] >52%) requiring phlebotomy or temporary cessation of testosterone therapy. No significant change in sleep-disordered breathing was reported, however.[18]

In a larger, randomized, placebo-controlled, cross-over trial of short-term high-dose T therapy, otherwise healthy participants with baseline T levels less than 450 ng/dL were given weekly injections of T (500 mg, 250 mg, 250 mg) and underwent polysomnographic testing and assessment of anthropometrics and airway bioimpedance. T treatment reduced rapid eye movement (REM) and non-REM (NREM) sleep by approximately 1 hour, although the proportion of time spent in each stage did not change significantly. RDI was increased by approximately 7 events per hour, and duration of hypoxemia was prolonged by T treatment. Interestingly, no significant change was seen in upper airway caliber, measured by awake acoustic reflectometry, or in neck and abdominal circumference. Rather, there was a reduction in serum leptin levels and adiposity, pointing to less pharyngeal fat deposition as a mechanism for the change in respiratory parameters.[19]

In a subsequent study, the same group studied obese adult men with OSA randomized to 3 intramuscular injections of T or placebo at 0, 6, and 12 weeks, and measured ventilatory chemoreflexes, including response to hypercapnea. They found a significant correlation between the hyperoxic carbon dioxide ventilatory recruitment threshold and increase in serum testosterone level at 6 weeks, indicating a dampened response to hypercapnea, along with a corresponding increase in time spent below oxygen saturation of 90% in sleep. A similar trend was seen for the ventilatory response in hypoxic conditions. This effect, however, did not persist on later measurements at week 18. The mechanism for this time-dependent difference in response remains to be better elucidated, although the findings suggest perhaps an effect of T on central chemoreceptors.[20]

MEN WITH OBSTRUCTIVE SLEEP APNEA AND SEXUAL DYSFUNCTION

There is growing evidence for an association between OSA and sexual dysfunction. Early observational data from Guilleminault and colleagues[21] indicated a high prevalence (48%) of erectile dysfunction (ED) in men with severe OSA. Margel and colleagues[22] also found a significant correlation between presence of ED and severe OSA, although the relationship was weaker in patients with mild or moderate disease. Composite results from a recent meta-analysis reported a relative risk of 1.82 for ED in men with OSA.[23]

EFFECT OF OBSTRUCTIVE SLEEP APNEA TREATMENT ON TESTOSTERONE LEVEL

The data investigating whether treating OSA results in an increase in T levels are mixed. One case series of 12 men with moderate-to-severe OSA who underwent uvulopalatopharyngoplasty (UPPP) showed small increases in T levels and improvement in self-reported sexual function 3 months after surgery without significant changes in prolactin, LH, or follicle-stimulating hormone (FSH) levels.[24] In another longitudinal study of 43 patients with severe OSA who were treated with nasal continuous positive airway pressure (CPAP), a significant increase in total T and sex hormone binding globulin (SHBG) was seen after 3 months of therapy, again suggesting a reversible component to the neuroendocrine dysfunction seen with OSA.[25] A randomized trial of 101 men with OSA who were given either therapeutic or sham CPAP showed that T and SHBG were negatively correlated to OSA severity at baseline. CPAP treatment did not increase T levels, but did result in SHBG elevation, along with increases in aldosterone and insulin-like growth factor 1 (IGF-1). The main drawback of this study was the short follow-up time of only 1 month.[25]

There are more positive data pointing to an improvement in sexual dysfunction with OSA treatment, independent of T levels. A study of 98 men with OSA found that those with ED had generally higher AHIs, lower oxygen saturation during sleep, and higher Epworth Sleepiness Scale and Beck Depression Inventory scores. These differences were eliminated with nasal CPAP treatment, and ED resolved in 75% of patients.[26] Another study that included over 200 patients also reported lower baseline T levels and International Index of Erectile Dysfuction-5 (IIEF-5) scores in men with severe OSA.[27] There were no significant differences in other hormones, including prolactin, LH, FSH, and estradiol. Three months of treatment with CPAP improved the IIEF-5 scores significantly, but did not result in changes in sexual hormone levels. Interestingly, a trial by Hoekema and colleagues[28] found no significant change in subjective measures of sexual function in a group of men with varying degrees of OSA when treated with either CPAP or an oral appliance.

In some of these patients with sexual dysfunction, there may be a benefit for using TRT. A pilot study evaluated TRT, PDE-5 inhibitor use, and CPAP in men with OSA and ED confirmed by nocturnal penile tumescence examination.[29] In the patients with normal T levels at baseline, use of a PDE-5 inhibitor alone was sufficient to correct ED (success rate >75%) after 6 months of therapy. However, in hypogonadal men, those treated with a combination of TRT, PDE-5 inhibitor, and CPAP did best, with normal erectile function after 3 months, compared with those who received PDE-5 inhibitor alone (only 42% showed improvement after 3 months). This suggests a positive additive benefit of TRT to PDE-5 inhibitors in hypogonadal men with OSA who receive CPAP therapy. It remains unclear whether TRT without CPAP would achieve a similar benefit. Larger, controlled studies are still needed.

OBSTRUCTIVE SLEEP APNEA AND POLYCYTHEMIA

Conditions of chronic hypoxemia, such as advanced lung disease and high altitude exposure, are known causes of polycythemia and cor pulmonale. OSA is characterized by repetitive periods of intermittent hypoxia, which has been proposed to be another risk factor for secondary polycythemia or erythrocytosis. Carlson and colleagues[30] described an increased prevalence of sleep-disordered breathing among patients with unexplained polycythemia in the absence of a difference in erythropoietin levels. In a larger study, Hoffstein and colleagues found a weak association between sleep apnea and increased Hct levels. Patients with more severe sleep apnea and longer periods of low nocturnal oxygen saturation (below 85%) appeared to have marginally higher Hct, although none reached polycythemic levels of Hct greater than 55%.[31] A subsequent investigation by Choi and colleagues found a significant correlation between Hct and respiratory disturbance index (RDI), another marker of OSA severity, mean oxygen saturation, and sleep time below oxygen saturation of 90%. Moreover, patients with severe OSA (RDI >30) had higher Hct than patients with mild-to-moderate disease (Hct 43.5% vs 41.2%), even after adjusting for gender, ethnicity, BMI, blood pressure, and catecholamine levels. Again, however, no clinically significant polycythemia was detected, suggesting that Hct is less useful as a screening tool for OSA.[32]

Up to 20% to 30% of patients with OSA also have concurrent obesity hypoventilation, characterized by chronic hypercapnia and sustained nocturnal hypoxemia.[33,34] Similar to patients with chronic obstructive pulmonary disease (COPD), secondary erythrocytosis has been described in patients with chronic alveolar hypoventilation, usually associated with states of prolonged hypoxemia.[35,36] It is possible that hypoxia-induced vascular growth factors play a role in this up-regulation of erythrocytes.[37] Therefore, evaluation for underlying causes of hypoventilation, in addition to OSA, is often recommended as part of the work-up for secondary polycythemia.[38] Importantly, this relationship should be kept in mind when considering the patient with OSA and hypogonadism who is considering T replacement, as T replacement is known to exacerbate polycythemia in some patients.

Interestingly, a few small studies have described a decrease in hematocrit levels with OSA treatment.[39] Krieger and colleagues measured Hct and red cell count before and after a single night of nasal CPAP therapy in a group of 8 patients with sleep apnea and found a small reduction in both parameters post-therapy (Hct 45.6% vs 43%). In a follow-up study, the same group tracked patients with unequivocal OSA (AHI >30/h) over the course of 1 year before and after CPAP therapy. They again found a decrease in Hct following just 1 night of CPAP therapy, with rebound effects seen off positive airway pressure. Hct remained in the range of the initial post-treatment baseline value on long-term follow-up (42.4% vs 42.9%). The mechanism of these effects remains unclear, with several hypotheses proposed, including fluid shifts and changes in red cell volume.[40,41]

SUMMARY

The relationships between T and OSA are complex and not yet completely understood. Available evidence points to reduced T levels in men with OSA, along with higher incidence of fatigue and sexual dysfunction. Some of the proposed mechanisms explaining this effect are alteration of sleep architecture, periods of low oxygen saturation in sleep, and changes in control hormone levels. There is concern that TRT, when given in high doses or alone without adequate treatment of OSA, may further compromise respiratory and polysomnographic parameters, with or without significant changes in airway dynamics. On the other hand, treatment of OSA may help improve sexual function, especially in men with severe disease. Additional systematic investigation of these clinically important questions is needed.

REFERENCES

1. Young T, Palta M, Dempsey J, et al. The occurrence of sleep-disordered breathing among middle-aged adults. N Engl J Med 1993;328:1230–5.
2. Nieto FJ, Young TB, Lind BK, et al. Association of sleep-disordered breathing, sleep apnea, and hypertension in a large community-based study: sleep heart health study. JAMA 2000;283:1829–36 [Erratum appears in JAMA 2002;288:1985].
3. Gottlieb DJ, Yenokyan G, Newman AB, et al. Prospective study of obstructive sleep apnea and incident coronary heart disease and heart failure: the sleep heart health study. Circulation 2010;122:352–60.
4. Redline S, Yenokyan G, Gottlieb DJ, et al. Obstructive sleep apnea–hypopnea and incident stroke: the sleep heart health study. Am J Respir Crit Care Med 2010;182:269–77.
5. Boyar RM, Rosenfeld RS, Kapen S, et al. Human puberty. simultaneous augmented secretion of luteinizing hormone and testosterone during sleep. J Clin Invest 1974;54(3):609–18.
6. Camargo CA. Obstructive sleep apnea and testosterone. N Engl J Med 1983;309(5):314–5.
7. Evans JI, MacLean AW, Ismail AA, et al. Concentrations of plasma testosterone in normal men during sleep. Nature 1971;229(5282):261–2.
8. Axelsson J, Ingre M, Akerstedt T, et al. Effects of acutely displaced sleep on testosterone. J Clin Endocrinol Metab 2005;90(8):4530–5.
9. Canguven O, Salepci B, Albayrak S, et al. Is there a correlation between testosterone levels and the severity of the disease in male patients with obstructive sleep apnea? Arch Ital Urol Androl 2010;82(4):143–7.
10. Gambineri A, Pelusi C, Pasquali R. Testosterone levels in obese male patients with obstructive sleep apnea syndrome: relation to oxygen desaturation, body weight, fat distribution and the metabolic parameters. J Endocrinol Invest 2003;26(6):493–8.
11. Hammoud AO, Walker JM, Gibson M, et al. Sleep apnea, reproductive hormones and quality of sexual life in severely obese men. Obesity (Silver Spring) 2011;19(6):1118–23.
12. Luboshitzky R, Lavie L, Shen-Orr Z, et al. Altered luteinizing hormone and testosterone secretion in middle-aged obese men with obstructive sleep apnea. Obes Res 2005;13(4):780–6.
13. Chervin R. Sleepiness, fatigue, tiredness, and lack of energy in obstructive sleep apnea. Chest 2000;118(2):372–9.
14. Bercea RM, Mihaescu T, Cojocaru C, et al. Fatigue and serum testosterone in obstructive sleep apnea patients. Clin Respir J 2015;9(3):342–9.
15. Cistulli PA, Grunstein RR, Sullivan CE. Effect of testosterone administration on upper airway collapsibility during sleep. Am J Respir Crit Care Med 1994;149(2 Pt 1):530–2.
16. Schneider BK, Pickett CK, Zwillich CW, et al. Influence of testosterone on breathing during sleep. J Appl Physiol (1985) 1986;61(2):618–23.

17. Matsumoto AM, Sandblom RE, Schoene RB, et al. Testosterone replacement in hypogonadal men: effects on obstructive sleep apnoea, respiratory drives, and sleep. Clin Endocrinol (Oxf) 1985; 22(6):713–21.

18. Hajjar RR, Kaiser FE, Morley JE. Outcomes of long-term testosterone replacement in older hypogonadal males: a retrospective analysis. J Clin Endocrinol Metab 1997;82(11):3793–6.

19. Liu PY, Yee B, Wishart SM, et al. The short-term effects of high-dose testosterone on sleep, breathing, and function in older men. J Clin Endocrinol Metab 2003;88(8):3605–13.

20. Killick R, Wang D, Hoyos CM, et al. The effects of testosterone on ventilatory responses in men with obstructive sleep apnea: a randomised, placebo-controlled trial. J Sleep Res 2013;22(3):331–6.

21. Guilleminault C, Simmons FB, Motta J, et al. Obstructive sleep apnea syndrome and tracheostomy. Long-term follow-up experience. Arch Intern Med 1981;141:985–8.

22. Margel D, Cohen M, Livne PM, et al. Severe, but not mild, obstructive sleep apnea syndrome is associated with erectile dysfunction. Urology 2004;63: 545–9.

23. Liu L, Kang R, Zhao S, et al. Sexual dysfunction in patients with obstructive sleep apnea: a systematic review and meta-analysis. J Sex Med 2015;12(10): 1992–2003.

24. Santamaria JD, Prior JC, Fleetham JA. Reversible reproductive dysfunction in men with obstructive sleep apnoea. Clin Endocrinol (Oxf) 1988;28(5): 461–70.

25. Grunstein RR, Handelsman DJ, Lawrence SJ, et al. Neuroendocrine dysfunction in sleep apnea: reversal by continuous positive airways pressure therapy. J Clin Endocrinol Metab 1989;68(2):352–8.

26. Goncalves MA, Guilleminault C, Ramos E, et al. Erectile dysfunction, obstructive sleep apnea syndrome and nasal CPAP treatment. Sleep Med 2005;6(4):333–9.

27. Zhang XB, Lin QC, Zeng HQ, et al. Erectile dysfunction and sexual hormone levels in men with obstructive sleep apnea: efficacy of continuous positive airway pressure. Arch Sex Behav 2015;45(1):235–40.

28. Hoekema A, Stel AL, Stegenga B, et al. Sexual function and obstructive sleep apnea-hypopnea: a randomized clinical trial evaluating the effects of oral-appliance and continuous positive airway pressure therapy. J Sex Med 2007;4:1153–62.

29. Zhuravlev VN, Frank MA, Gomzhin AI. Sexual functions of men with obstructive sleep apnoea syndrome and hypogonadism may improve upon testosterone administration: a pilot study. Andrologia 2009;41(3):193–5.

30. Carlson JT, Hedner J, Fagerberg B, et al. Secondary polycythaemia associated with nocturnal apnoea–a relationship not mediated by erythropoietin? J Intern Med 1992;231(4):381–7.

31. Hoffstein V, Herridge M, Mateika S, et al. Hematocrit levels in sleep apnea. Chest 1994;106(3):787–91.

32. Choi JB, Loredo JS, Norman D, et al. Does obstructive sleep apnea increase hematocrit? Sleep Breath 2006;10:155–6.

33. Dabal L, BaHamman AS. Obesity hypoventilation syndrome. Ann Thorac Med 2009;4(2):41–9.

34. Mokhlesi B, Tulaimat A, Faibussowitsch I, et al. Obesity hypoventilation syndrome: prevalence and predictors in patients with obstructive sleep apnea. Sleep Breath 2007;11(2):117–24.

35. Lawrence T. Idiopathic hypoventilation, polycythemia, and cor pulmonale. Am Rev Respir Dis 1959;80(4):575–81.

36. Kent BD, Mitchell PD, McNicholas WT. Hypoxemia in patients with COPD: cause, effects, and disease progression. Int J Chron Obstruct Pulmon Dis 2011;6:199–208.

37. Semenza GL. Regulation of oxygen homeostasis by hypoxia-inducible factor 1. Physiology 2009;24: 97–106.

38. Lee G, Arcasoy MO. The clinical and laboratory evaluation of the patient with erythrocytosis. Eur J Intern Med 2015;26(5):297–302.

39. Krieger J, Sforza E, Delanoe C, et al. Decrease in hematocrit with continuous positive airway pressure treatment in obstructive sleep apnea patients. Eur Respir J 1992;5:228–33.

40. Saarelainen S, Hasan J, Seppala E. Effect of nasal CPAP treatment on plasma volume, aldosterone and 24-h blood pressure in obstructive sleep apnea. J Sleep Res 1996;5:181–5.

41. Krieger J, Follenius M, Sforza E, et al. Effects of treatment with nasal continuous positive airway pressure on atrial natriuretic peptide and arginine vasopressin release during sleep in obstructive sleep apnea. Clin Sci 1991;80:443–9.

Assessing and Managing Sleep Disturbance in Patients with Chronic Pain

Martin D. Cheatle, PhD[a,b,*], Simmie Foster, MD, PhD[c],
Aaron Pinkett, BS[a], Matthew Lesneski, MD[d],
David Qu, MD[e], Lara Dhingra, PhD[f]

KEYWORDS

- Chronic pain • Insomnia • Cognitive behavior therapy • Sleep-disordered breathing
- Pharmacotherapy

KEY POINTS

- Sleep disturbance is common in patients with chronic pain (CP).
- Sleep and pain are bidirectional; pain can interfere with sleep and sleep disturbance can exacerbate pain.
- The presence of sleep-disordered breathing, including obstructive sleep apnea and central sleep apnea, increases the risk of significant harm associated with the use of opioids and other centrally sedating medications.
- Cognitive behavior therapy (CBT) has the potential to improve both pain and sleep quality.
- There are several pharmacologic agents used to improve sleep disturbance in the CP population.

INTRODUCTION

Patients with CP often present to clinicians with numerous medical and psychological comorbidities, including mood and anxiety disorders, secondary medical problems related to inactivity and weight gain, and sleep disturbance. Insomnia can be generally defined as the inability to acquire adequate sleep to feel rested in the morning. Insomnia can be due to difficulties initiating or maintaining sleep or both. Chronic insomnia (occurring at least 3 times per week for at least 3 months) usually leads to daytime consequences, such as fatigue, reduced mental acuity, and so forth.

It has been estimated that the prevalence of sleep disturbance in patients with CP ranges between 50% and 80%.[1–5] For example, Tang and colleagues[1] evaluated 70 patients with chronic back pain and compared them to 70 gender-matched and age-matched pain-free control patients, measuring sleep disturbance, pain, and a variety of psychological variables, including health

This article originally appeared in *Anesthesiology Clinics*, Volume 34, Issue 2, June 2016.
Conflicts of Interest: None of the authors has any conflicts of interest related to the material in this article.
[a] Department of Psychiatry, Center for Studies of Addiction, Perelman School of Medicine, University of Pennsylvania, 3535 Market Street, 4th Floor, Philadelphia, PA 19104, USA; [b] Department of Psychiatry, Behavioral Medicine Center, Reading Health System, 560 Van Reed Road, Suite 204, Wyomissing, PA 19610, USA; [c] Kirby Center for Neurobiology, 3 Blackfan Circle, CLS 12-260, Boston, MA 02115, USA; [d] RA Pain Services, 1500 Midatlantic Drive Suite 102, Mount Laurel, NJ 0854, USA; [e] Highpoint Pain and Rehabilitation Physicians P.C., 700 Horizon Circle Suite 206, Chalfont, PA 18914, USA; [f] MJHS Institute for Innovation in Palliative Care, 39 Broadway, 3rd Floor, New York, NY 10006, USA
* Corresponding author. Center for Studies of Addiction, Perelman School of Medicine, University of Pennsylvania, 3535 Market Street, 4th Floor, Philadelphia, PA 19104.
E-mail address: cheatle@mail.med.upenn.edu

status anxiety and depression. Results indicated that 53% of the patients with CP demonstrated evidence of clinical insomnia, with only 3% of the pain-free controls meeting criteria for insomnia. Furthermore, insomnia severity was positively associated with pain intensity, sensory pain ratings, affective pain ratings, general anxiety, general depression, and health anxiety. Affective pain ratings and health status anxiety were the best predictors of insomnia severity, which suggests that emotional distress is strongly linked to sleep disturbance. In another study by McCracken and colleagues,[2] 159 patients undergoing evaluation at a pain management center were assessed for history of sleep disturbance. In this cohort, 79% met criteria for significant insomnia based on self-reported symptoms.

There is persuasive evidence to support the hypothesis that the association between pain and sleep are bidirectional in nature.[6,7] Sivertsen and colleagues[7] collected data on CP and sleep and assessed experimental pain sensitivity via cold pressor testing in 10,412 adults in Norway. The results of this study revealed that insomnia frequency and severity, sleep-onset problems, and sleep efficiency were positively associated with pain sensitivity. Results also revealed that pain tolerance was reduced further in a synergistic fashion in subjects who reported both CP and insomnia. Clinical studies have proved that CP patients who reported sleep disturbance also note increased pain, more fatigue, poor mood, and generally higher levels of stress and disability.[8,9] Experimental studies in healthy controls demonstrate that sleep deprivation or disruption leads to an increase in pain via an increase in the release of proinflammatory cytokines[10] and a decrease in pain tolerance.[11] There has also been some speculation that pain, sleep, and depression share underlying neurobiological mechanisms.[12]

Despite the burgeoning evidence for the bidirectional association between pain and sleep and the deleterious effects of sleep deprivation on mood, pain sensitivity, and disability, addressing sleep disturbance in patients with CP is often overlooked in the clinical encounter due to the many competing concerns. The aim of this article is to provide clinicians with a basic understanding of assessing sleep disturbance and the use of nonpharmacologic and pharmacologic treatment strategies to improve sleep quality in patients with CP. This article does not include a discussion of other sleep disorders, in particular, sleep-disordered breathing (obstructive sleep apnea and central sleep apnea). It is critical to assess and monitor obstructive sleep apnea and central sleep apnea in patients considered for opioid therapy or who

are receiving opioids, because a significant percentage of patients on opioid therapy has sleep-disordered breathing. A recently published article by Cheatle and Webster[13] specifically addresses the topic of sleep-disordered breathing and opioids in patients with CP.

ASSESSMENT OF SLEEP DISTURBANCE

Polysomnography (PSG) and self-report measures of sleep disturbance are standard approaches used in insomnia research. More recently, actigraphy has been used as an objective measure of sleep quality in sleep research. There are also several commercially available activity-sleep monitors that can be used clinically in assessing and monitoring sleep duration. Self-report questionnaires are more commonly used because they

1. Are inexpensive
2. Are the primary assessment tool used by clinicians treating insomnia
3. Standardize methods across research studies given the lack of a biomarker for insomnia and a universally accepted definition of insomnia[14]

The selection of a self-report measure depends on a clinician's goals. These goals may vary from screening and diagnosis to monitoring of previously identified sleep disturbances to evaluating the efficacy of treatment interventions. There are several sleep assessment scales that evaluate multiple dimensions of sleep, including sleep quality, sleep onset, postsleep evaluation, and generic outcomes. Of these, sleep quality and postsleep evaluation measures are the most commonly used. Examples of various sleep instruments are outlined in **Table 1**.[15–20] Moul and colleagues[14] also provide a comprehensive review of the different sleep scales.

Each measure has varying degrees of utility depending on the nature of the sleep disturbance, the level of severity, and the specific characteristics of sleep a clinician seeks to assess. It is important to select a sleep instrument that fits the dynamics of the clinical setting, such as time constraints, patient burden, and staff resources.

NONPHARMACOLOGIC INTERVENTIONS
Cognitive Behavior Therapy for Pain and Sleep

Medications are commonly used to manage both pain and insomnia; however, the use of medications can result in adverse effects, dependence, and poor treatment efficacy. The use of nonpharmacologic approaches for pain and insomnia may mitigate these negative effects, but clinicians seldom implement psychological strategies.

Table 1
Self-report measures for assessment of insomnia

Domain	Scale	Time Frame	No. of Items	Comments
Postsleep evaluation	Wolff's Morning Questions[15]	Today	8	Yes/no questions detailing morning restedness, presence of bedpartner, etc.
Postsleep evaluation	Kryger's Subjective Measurements[16]	Today	9	Mixed format questions detailing sleep onset, sleep latency, etc.
Postsleep evaluation	Morning Sleep Questionnaire[17]	Today	4	Mixed format questions evaluating sleep goodness and other factors
Sleep quality	Pittsburgh Sleep Quality Index[18]	Past month	24	Mixed format questions and household-related questions that use an algorithm to score sleep disturbance
Sleep quality	Sleep Questionnaire[19]	Indefinite	59	Questions use Likert-type scale responses ranging from sleep depth to dream recall/vividness
Sleep quality	Sleep Disturbance Questionnaire[20]	Indefinite	12	Questions use Likert-type scale responses that assess mental anxiety and physical tension

Data from Refs.[15–20]

Evidence-based CBT approaches for pain (CBT-P) and for insomnia (CBT-I) are well developed, efficacious, and cost effective and may improve clinical outcomes and treatment response for different subpopulations with varied pain conditions. Many clinicians lack training in the effective use of CBT techniques, however, or there is poor access to these services.

Cognitive behavior therapy for pain
A variety of psychological and behavioral strategies are effective for CP management, including CBT, acceptance and commitment therapy, mindfulness-based stress reduction, progressive muscle relaxation training, motivational interviewing, and goal setting to increase behavioral activation.[21–23] CBT may incorporate any of these specific components. CBT techniques usually involve the identification of maladaptive or dysfunctional thoughts and behaviors that may worsen patient adjustment to CP and disability. The evaluation and modification of negative thought patterns and their substitution with more rational cognitions can reframe patients' interpretations that contribute to feelings of suffering, demoralization, and helplessness. CBT may assist patients in developing and implementing specific strategies, such as progressive muscle relaxation train, activity pacing, distraction techniques, and positive self-talk, to help them cope with negative affect caused by pain and disability.

CBT-P has been shown highly effective at reducing patient distress in a variety of pain disorders.[24–27] It might be expected that improved pain

would translate into improved sleep for patients. It is difficult, however, to make this conclusion because few studies evaluating the efficacy of CBT-P in a CP population have examined sleep. Although the data are inconclusive, the few studies that included sleep measures suggested minimal improvement in sleep after CBT-P.[28,29] Based on this observation, CP patients suffering from insomnia may achieve the most improvement in sleep from interventions that specifically target sleep disturbance.

Cognitive behavior therapy for insomnia
In studies of patients with chronic primary insomnia, CBT-I has been shown equally effective or even superior to pharmacotherapy in multiple outcomes. Sivertsen and colleagues[30] compared CBT-I to standard therapy with eszopiclone and found that the CBT-I treatment group had increased time spent in slow-wave restorative sleep and improved sleep efficiency (proportion of time spent in bed actually sleeping).

A course of CBT-I typically consists of

- Psychoeducation about sleep and insomnia
- Stimulus control
- Sleep restriction
- Sleep hygiene
- Relaxation training
- Cognitive therapy

Stimulus control strengthens a patient's association of the bed with rapid-onset sleep, by teaching the patient to limit the use of bed to sex and sleep, avoid daytime naps, maintain a regular sleep/wake time, go to bed only when sleepy, and get out of bed if not asleep within 15 to 20 minutes. Sleep restriction limits the amount of time a patient spends in bed to the actual time asleep, so, for example, if a patient spends 8 hours in bed but only 4 hours total asleep, the patient is instructed to spend only 4 hours in bed. This leads initially to a mild sleep deprivation, which increases the patient's drive to sleep and leads to more consolidated, restful sleep and greater sleep efficiency. Over time, as sleep efficiency improves, the patient gradually increases time in bed. Sleep hygiene increases patients' awareness of behavioral and environmental factors that have an impact on sleep, such as how caffeine, alcohol, periods of intense exercise, bright lights, and use of electronic devices before bed may be detrimental to sleep, as well as education on the benefits of a restful bedroom environment. Relaxation training reduces cognitive and physical tension close to bedtime and involves techniques, such as hypnosis, meditation, and guided imagery. Cognitive therapy helps patients explore how beliefs and attitudes toward sleep affect sleep behaviors. Patients learn to identify maladaptive or distorted thoughts and replace them with more adaptive substitutes, thereby helping to alleviate worrying or rumination about insomnia.

CBT-I has been shown in several studies to improve sleep in patients with CP. For example, Jungquist and colleagues,[31] in a study of 28 patients with chronic back and neck pain, found that those patients who received CBT-I had significantly improved sleep and maintained improvements in total sleep time at 6 months post-treatment completion, despite the persistence of moderate to severe pain.

Combined treatment of pain and sleep

Given the effectiveness of CBT-I and of CBT-P, there has been growing interest in the feasibility of combining CBT-I with CBT-P. In a small pilot study of 20 patients with CP, Tang and colleagues[32] found that a hybrid CBT-I/CBT-P intervention was associated with greater improvement in sleep at post-treatment. Although pain intensity did not change, the hybrid group reported greater reductions in pain interference, fatigue, and depression than the controls, and overall changes were clinically significant and durable at 1-month and 6-month follow-ups. Thus current evidence suggests that CBT is an important treatment that should be used in the treatment of insomnia in CP patients.

PHARMACOTHERAPY

For many patients with CP, uncontrolled pain precipitates sleep and mood disturbance, so naturally clinicians often first focus exclusively on treating pain.[33] Due to the reciprocal relationship between pain and sleep, however, it is important to concurrently treat sleep disorders; pharmacologic treatments aimed at improvements in sleep have been shown to decrease pain intensity.[34,35] Given the complex presentation of patients with CP and sleep disturbance, clinicians usually tailor pharmacologic therapy for insomnia based on a patients pain pathophysiology and comorbid conditions. The most commonly used medications for insomnia are reviewed and their role for patients with CP and sleep disturbance highlighted. An overview of pharmacologic sleep agents, dosing, and adverse effects is in **Table 2**.

Opioid Analgesics

Several studies have shown that opioid medications may improve subjective quality of sleep; for example, 1 study in patients with osteoarthritis found that extended-release morphine sulfate was associated with improvements in objective sleep measures of PSG, including sleep efficiency.[36] In contrast, there have also been studies that demonstrate that opioids can inhibit both rapid eye movement and non–rapid eye movement sleep, contributing to an exacerbation of pain.[37,38] There is also compelling evidence that long-term use of opioid analgesics may lead to adverse effects, including sleep-disordered breathing, opioid-induced hyperalgesia, tolerance, and dependence in populations at risk.[39] Therefore, although opioids may be effective in carefully selected patients for the treatment of pain, opioids should never be used to treat insomnia.

Benzodiazepine Receptor Agonists

Benzodiazepine receptor agonists (BzRAS) include benzodiazepines (eg, temazepam and triazolam) and the newer class of nonbenzodiazepine drugs (eg, zolpidem and eszopiclone). This class of drugs binds to γ-aminobutyric acid (GABA)-A receptors and induces sedative/hypnotic, amnestic, anxiolytic, muscle relaxant, and anticonvulsant effects.[40,41] Many short-term clinical trials show that BzRAs improve sleep quality, sleep latency, wakefulness after sleep onset, and total sleep time.[40] Most benzodiazepines (excluding triazolam) have intermediate to long half-lives and, therefore, may help patients fall asleep and stay asleep.

Food and Drug Administration (FDA)-approved benzodiazepines for insomnia include temazepam, triazolam, estazolam, quazepam, and flurazepam.[42] Lorazepam, alprazolam, and clonazepam are anxiolytics that are often used off-label for sleep.

Table 2
Pharmacologic sleep agents, dosing, and adverse effects

Agent	Dose	Adverse Effects	Comments
Amitriptyline	10–100 mg	Orthostatic hypotension, daytime sedation, anticholinergic effects, cardiac conduction abnormality, sexual dysfunction, weight gain	Used for neuropathic pain, tension headaches, and fibromyalgia
Doxepin	3–6 mg proprietary, 10–100 mg generic	Minimal anticholinergic side effects at hypnotic doses	FDA approved for insomnia
Mirtazapine	7.5–30 mg	Increased appetite, weight gain, anticholinergic effects	Excellent for patients with poor appetite, mood and sleep disturbance
Trazodone	25–100 mg	Dizziness, anticholinergic effects, daytime sedation, priapism, neuropathic pain	May be helpful in diabetic neuropathy and fibromyalgia
Temazepam	15–50 mg	Sedation, fatigue, depression, dizziness, ataxia, confusion	FDA approved for insomnia; no evidence for long-term use
Clonazepam	0.5–3 mg	Sedation, fatigue, depression, dizziness, ataxia, confusion	Used for restless leg syndrome, anxiety, muscle spasm, anticonvulsant activity. May be beneficial for patients with neuropathic pain; no evidence or long-term use for sleep
Zolpidem	5–10 mg (immediate release) 6.25–12.5 mg (extended release)	Aberrant sleep-related behaviors	Most prescribed hypnotic
Zaleplon	5–20 mg	—	Shortest active BzRA; useful for patients with nocturnal awakenings
Eszopiclone	1–03 mg	Unpleasant taste, sedation, dizziness	Well tolerated; may boost antidepressant and anxiolytic efficacy
Melatonin	0.5–3 mg	—	Well tolerated; over-the-counter no FDA approval; useful for shift workers/delayed sleep phase
Ramelteon	8 mg	—	FDA approved; few adverse effects other than sedation, main effect on sleep latency
Quetiapine	25–50 mg	Dry mouth, weight gain, metabolic syndromes, orthostatic hypotension rare dystonias	Effective in anxiety disorders
Gabapentin	100–900 mg	Dizziness, ataxia, fatigue, weight gain, lower extremity swelling	Used for neuropathic pain, fibromyalgia with comorbid sleep disturbance
Diphenhydramine	25–50 mg	Anticholinergic side effects	Caution with elderly, no literature to support chronic use, no evidence for pain control

For patients with CP, short-term use of benzodiazepines may be useful in improving muscle tension, anxiety, and neuropathic pain as well as sleep.[43,44] One early study found, however, that with long-term use (>1 year), pain patients using benzodiazepines reported no significant clinical improvements in sleep.[45]

Although the benzodiazepines may work well in short-term efficacy trials, few data are available on long-term use, and there are many documented adverse effects. In the elderly, standard doses may lead to ataxia and psychomotor impairment, which may increase the risk of falls and hip fractures.[46] All BzRAs can cause cognitive impairment and decreased attention, specifically anterograde amnesia.[47] Long-term use of benzodiazepines may increase depressive symptomatology, with cognitive and psychomotor slowing.[45] In addition, abruptly stopping the drug may lead to rebound insomnia and seizures. There is also a concern of tolerance and dependence, especially in patients with a history of sedative or alcohol abuse.[48]

Care should be taken to not use more than 1 benzodiazepine at once (for example, temazepam for sleep and clonazepam for muscle relaxation), because many drugs in this class have active metabolites that can combine and lead to delayed sedation.[40] Also, the use of benzodiazepines in combination with opioids presents increased risk of harm to patients, especially those patients with sleep-disordered breathing. In addition, combining opioids with benzodiazepines should be avoided in patients with depression, especially in those patients with suicidal ideation.

Nonbenzodiazepine Benzodiazepine Receptor Agonists

The nonbenzodiazepine BzRAs (NBzRAs), zolpidem, zaleplon, and eszopiclone, are the newest class of FDA-approved hypnotics used for insomnia. They universally improve sleep latency and have the potential for fewer daytime side effects give their shorter half-lives and receptor binding profile. Long-term efficacy trials have supported their use.[49,50]

Zolpidem is currently the most widely prescribed drug for insomnia. In contrast to the benzodiazepines, 1 double-blind, placebo-controlled study showed that nightly use of zolpidem remained effective after 8 months of nightly use with no evidence of tolerance or rebound effects.[50]

Eszopiclone was approved by the FDA for the treatment of insomnia with no short-term restrictions on use. Similar to zolpidem, studies suggest that eszopiclone is effective for 6 to 12 months of long-term use.[51] In addition, eszopiclone augments the effects of antidepressants and anxiolytics in patients who have insomnia and comorbid depression or anxiety.[49]

The use of both zolpidem and eszopiclone is associated with improved sleep and quality of life in fibromyalgia and rheumatoid arthritis patients.[44,52,53] In terms of safety, similar to triazolam, zolpidem and zaleplon are associated with sleep-related behaviors, including sleep eating, sleep walking, and sleep driving.[40] For zolpidem, recent data on cognitive function and drug blood levels have prompted the FDA to lower the recommended daily dose for women.[40] In contrast to studies of typical benzodiazepines, recent studies of zolpidem, zaleplon, and eszoplicone have not noted tolerance or discontinuation effects. Although there are limited and conflicting data on the potential risk of this class of medications on sleep-disordered breathing[54] there is some evidence that NBzRAS have contributed to deaths, typically in combination with other central nervous system depressants, including opioids.[55] Clinicians should consider the potential added risk of prescribing NBzRAS to patients with CP receiving opioids and alternatively use medications for insomnia with a lower risk profile.

Antidepressants

Sedative antidepressants, such as tricyclic antidepressants (TCAs), mirtazapine, and trazodone, are useful in treating CP patients with insomnia by helping to relieve

1. Insomnia
2. Depressive symptoms that likely enhance pain perception
3. The pain condition itself[33]

TCAs (amitriptyline, nortriptyline, desipramine, clomipramine, imipramine, trimipramine, and doxepin) have proserotonergic, noradrenergic, dopaminergic, and sodium-channel blocking effects that may account for their efficacy in pain and depression, along with anticholinergic and antihistaminic effects that lead to sedation. At standard doses, all TCAs have shown equal efficacy in treating neuropathic pain; however, they are not all equal in promoting sleep.[56,57] For example, desipramine and imipramine are less sedating and may disrupt sleep.[58,59] Amitriptyline, nortriptyline, trimipramine, and doxepin, on the other hand, may decrease sleep latency, increase sleep efficiency, and increase total sleep time.[56,60]

Amitriptyline is probably the best studied TCA for improving sleep in patients with comorbid pain, especially headache, fibromyalgia, and neuropathic pain.[61–63] It may be poorly tolerated, however, due to anticholinergic side effects. Nortriptyline, a metabolite of amitriptyline, may cause less sedation but may also have fewer side effects, including less daytime drowsiness.[64]

Doxepin, the only TCA approved by the FDA for the treatment of insomnia, has a hypnotic dose of 1 mg to 6 mg as opposed to 150 mg to 300 mg when used as an antidepressant. At the lower doses, doxepin is selective for histamine type 1 receptors, which may explain its sedative effects without typical anticholinergic adverse effects. Safety and efficacy studies revealed reduced wakefulness after sleep onset, increased sleep efficiency, and total sleep time without next-day sedation or anticholinergic effects.[65] At these doses, doxepin has not been formally studied for an analgesic or antidepressant effect, although it may be titrated as tolerated to improve pain syndromes.[41]

Adverse effects of TCAs, due to anti–α-adrenergic and anticholinergic effects, include orthostatic hypotension, dry mouth and eyes, constipation, and cardiac conduction delays. In addition, TCAs may prolong the QT interval, leading to increased risk for serious cardiac arrhythmias. Risks of cardiac-related adverse effects, including orthostatic hypotension, increase with increased age. The blood levels of TCAs can be increased by the concurrent use of several medications, including selective serotonin reuptake inhibitors. Because the risk for serious adverse events is increased with increased TCA blood levels, care must be taken to carefully consider concurrent medications and make appropriate dose adjustments when indicated. Clinicians must also be cautious when prescribing TCAs to depressed and suicidal patients, because they are extremely lethal in overdose (lethality may occur with as little as 1 g).[66]

Trazodone is an antagonist of serotonin type 2, histamine, and α_1-adrenergic receptors, and mildly inhibits serotonin reuptake. Similar to the other antidepressants, trazodone exerts most of its hypnotic effects at low doses and has antidepressant effects at higher doses. Several studies show that trazodone improves sleep in the elderly, depressed patients, and patients with anxiety disorders and posttraumatic stress disorder.[67] Trazodone has also been studied in patients with various pain syndromes, including fibromyalgia and diabetic neuropathy, where it was associated with both improved pain and sleep quality.[68,69] There is also some evidence for adjunctive effects when used with pregabalin for CP patients.[67] There are concerns about tolerance with this drug, however; in 1 study trazodone was shown

as effective as zolpidem on sleep latency and total sleep time but only during the first 2 weeks of therapy.[70] Side effects include next-day drowsiness, rebound insomnia, orthostatic hypotension, dry mouth, and, rarely, priapism.

Mirtazapine is an antidepressant with sedating qualities due to the antagonism of type 1 histaminergic and serotonin type 2 receptors. At doses of 15 mg to 30 mg, it improves sleep latency, total sleep time, and sleep efficiency and decreases frequency of night awakenings.[56] It has been shown to improve sleep, pain, appetite, and mood in cancer patients.[71] In addition, several studies have suggested that mirtazapine is useful for the treatment of pain caused by recurrent headache and postherpetic neuralgia.[72–74]

Selective serotonin reuptake inhibitors and serotonin-norepinephrine reuptake inhibitors (SNRIs), although effective for depression and pain, have been shown to disrupt and fragment sleep.[60] Duloxetine, an SNRI, is often used to treat neuropathic pain and comorbid mood but has been shown to decrease sleep efficiency.[33,61] Dosing of the SNRI during the day and avoiding SNRI use in the evening hours may help to mitigate this adverse effect.

Antipsychotics

Two of the newer atypical antipsychotic medications, quetiapine and olanzapine, are used off-label for the treatment of insomnia. Self-reported outcomes and PSG data suggest efficacy in increasing total sleep time and slow wave restorative sleep and in decreasing sleep latency.[64,75] At low doses, quetiapine primarily has antihistiminergic properties and is weakly proserotonergic. It has been shown to decrease anxiety and enhance the effects of antidepressant medication.[64] In addition, several case reports and open-label studies show that quetiapine and olanzapine have analgesic properties, especially for fibromyalgia and migraine disorders.[75,76] These medications may cause significant weight gain (olanzapine more so than quetiapine), however. Cardiac conduction abnormalities (such as prolonged QT interval) should be monitored in patients using these drugs. In addition, there is a small risk of movement disorders, such as akathisia and tardive dyskinesia. If atypical antipsychotics are considered, it is advisable to do so in consultation with a psychiatrist.

Anticonvulsants

Gabapentin and pregabalin are GABA analogs often used to treat CP conditions with comorbid insomnia.[33] Across multiple studies of patients with neuropathic pain and fibromyalgia, self-reported sleep outcomes suggest positive effects on sleep latency and wakefulness after sleep onset as well as increased deep sleep.[33,77,78] Both drugs also have adjunctive effects on depression and anxiety.[79] A recent study showed that pregabalin was more effective in improving sleep among patients with diabetic neuropathy compared with amitriptyline.[61] Common adverse effects include dizziness, next-day sedation, gastrointestinal symptoms, and peripheral edema.

Over-the-Counter Medications

Melatonin receptor agonists include the natural ligand melatonin as well as nonmelatonin drugs such as ramelteon. Melatonin has been shown to induce sleep by attenuating the wake-promoting impulses in the suprachiasmatic nucleus of the hypothalamus. Melatonin is available over the counter and is not FDA approved. In 2005, the FDA approved ramelteon, a melatonin receptor agonist, for the treatment of sleep-onset insomnia. Both melatonin and ramelteon have mild efficacy for reducing sleep latency, especially in patients who have delayed sleep phases (sleep and wake times shifted later).[80] This population frequently includes older adults and shift workers. There is some evidence that melatonin may have analgesic effects in patients with fibromyalgia, irritable bowel syndrome, and migraine disorders.[81]

Most other over-the-counter sleep agents contain first-generation antihistamines, such as diphenhydramine and doxylamine, which also have anticholinergic effects. Diphenhydramine is the most commonly used nonprescription sleep aid. Patients, however, may quickly develop tolerance. To date there are no controlled trials that demonstrate the efficacy of diphenhydramine for greater than 3 weeks in the treatment of insomnia. Antihistamines can cause next-day sedation and impair cognitive function and should be used with caution in the elderly.

SUMMARY

Sleep disturbance commonly occurs in patients with CP and can cause additional distress and fatigue and may exacerbate pain. There is persuasive evidence that pain and sleep have a bidirectional relationship; pain can cause sleep disturbance and sleep disturbance can increase pain. Typically, sleep disturbance is not systematically evaluated, treated, and monitored in busy pain care settings. There are multiple evidenced-based nonpharmacologic and pharmacologic approaches that can significantly improve both sleep disturbance and co-occurring pain, and some may reduce the use of opioids in specific patients on long-term opioid therapy. The assessment of the multiple dimensions of sleep and basic treatment strategies should be incorporated into the routine care of patients with CP and included in pain education and training for professionals.

REFERENCES

1. Tang NK, Wright KJ, Salkovskis PM. Prevalence and correlates of clinical insomnia co-occurring with chronic back pain. J Sleep Res 2007;16(1):85–95.
2. McCracken LM, Williams JL, Tang NK. Psychological flexibility may reduce insomnia in persons with chronic pain: a preliminary retrospective study. Pain Med 2011;12(6):904–12.
3. Allen KD, Renner JB, DeVellis B, et al. Osteoarthritis and sleep: the Johnston County Osteoarthritis Project. J Rheumatol 2008;35:1102–7.
4. Artner J, Cakir B, Spiekermann JA, et al. Prevalence of sleep deprivation in patients with chronic neck and back pain: a retrospective evaluation of 1016 patients. J Pain Res 2013;6:1–6.
5. Alsaadi SM, McAuley JH, Hush JM, et al. Prevalence of sleep disturbance in patients with low back pain. Eur Spine J 2011;20(5):737–43.
6. Koffel E, Kroenke K, Bair MJ, et al. The bidirectional relationship between sleep complaints and pain: analysis of data from a randomized trial. Health Psychol 2016;35(1):41–9.
7. Sivertsen B, Lallukka T, Petrie KJ, et al. Sleep and pain sensitivity in adults. Pain 2015;156(8):1433–9.
8. Haythornthwaite JA, Hegel MT, Kerns RD. Development of a sleep diary for chronic pain patients. J Pain Symptom Manage 1991;6(2):65–72.
9. Chiu YH, Silman AJ, Macfarlane GJ, et al. Poor sleep and depression are independently associated with a reduced pain threshold. Results of a population based study. Pain 2005;115(3):316–21.
10. Moldofsky H, Lue FA, Eisen J, et al. The relationship of interleukin-1 and immune functions to sleep in humans. Psychosom Med 1986;48(5):309–18.
11. Onen SH, Alloui A, Gross A, et al. The effects of total sleep deprivation, selective sleep interruption and sleep recovery on pain tolerance thresholds in healthy subjects. J Sleep Res 2001;10(1):35–42.
12. Boakye PA, Olechowski C, Rashiq S, et al. A critical review of neurobiological factors involved in the interactions between chronic pain, depression, and sleep disruption. Clin J Pain 2015. [Epub ahead of print].
13. Cheatle MD, Webster LR. Opioid therapy and sleep disorders: risks and mitigation strategies. Pain Med 2015;16(Suppl 1):S22–6.
14. Moul DE, Hall M, Pilkonis PA, et al. Self-report measures of insomnia in adults: rationales, choices, and needs. Sleep Med Rev 2004;8(3):177–98.

15. Wolff BB. Evaluation of hypnotics in outpatients with insomnia using a questionnaire and a self-rating technique. Clin Pharmacol Ther 1974;15(2):130–40.

16. Kryger MH, Steljes D, Pouliot Z, et al. Subjective versus objective evaluation of hypnotic efficacy: experience with zolpidem. Sleep 1991;14(5):399–407.

17. Mendelson WB, Maczaj M. Effects of triazolam on the perception of wakefulness in insomniacs. Ann Clin Psychiatry 1990;2:211–5.

18. Buysse DJ, Reynolds CF 3rd, Monk TH, et al. The Pittsburgh Sleep Quality Index: a new instrument for psychiatric practice and research. Psychiatry Res 1989;28(2):193–213.

19. Domino G, Blair G, Bridges A. Subjective assessment of sleep by Sleep Questionnaire. Percept Mot Skills 1984;59(1):163–70.

20. Espie CA, Brooks DN, Lindsay WR. An evaluation of tailored psychological treatment of insomnia. J Behav Ther Exp Psychiatry 1989;20(2):143–53.

21. McCracken LM, Turk TC. Behavioral and cognitive-behavioral treatment for chronic pain: outcome, predictors of outcome, and treatment process. Spine (Phila Pa 1976) 2002;27(22):2564.

22. McCracken LM, Eccleston C, Vowles KE. Acceptance-based treatment for persons with complex, long standing chronic pain: a preliminary analysis of treatment outcome in comparison to a waiting phase. Behav Res Ther 2005;43:1335–46.

23. Williams AC, Eccleston C, Morley S. Psychological therapies for the management of chronic pain (excluding headache) in adults. Cochrane Database Syst Rev 2012;(11):CD007407.

24. Keefe FJ, Caldwell DS. Cognitive behavioral control of arthritis pain. Med Clin North Am 1997;81:277–90.

25. Glombiewski JA, Hartwich-Tersek J, Rief W. Two psychological interventions are effective in severely disabled, chronic back pain patients: a randomized controlled trial. Int J Behav Med 2010;17(2):97–107.

26. Turner JA, Manci L, Aaron LA. Short- and long-term efficacy of brief cognitive-behavioral therapy for patients with chronic tempromandibular disorder pain: a randomized, controlled trial. Pain 2006;121(3): 181–94.

27. Thieme K, Flor H, Turk D. Psychological pain treatment in fibromyalgia syndrome: efficacy of operant behavioral and cognitive behavioral treatments. Arthritis Res Ther 2006;8(4):R121.

28. Becker N, Sjøgren P, Bech P, et al. Treatment outcome of chronic non-malignant pain patients managed in a Danish multidisciplinary pain centre compared to general practice: a randomized controlled trial. Pain 2000;84(2–3):203–11.

29. Tang NK. Cognitive-behavioral therapy for sleep abnormalities of chronic pain patients. Curr Rheumatol Rep 2009;11(6):451–60.

30. Sivertsen B, Omvik S, Pallesen S, et al. Cognitive behavioral therapy vs zopiclone for treatment of chronic primary insomnia in older adults: a randomized controlled trial. JAMA 2006;295(24):2851–8.

31. Jungquist CR, Tra Y, Smith MT, et al. The durability of cognitive behavioral therapy for insomnia in patients with chronic pain. Sleep Disord 2012;2012:679648.

32. Tang NK, Goodchild CE, Salkovskis PM. Hybrid cognitive-behavior therapy for individuals with insomnia and chronic pain: a pilot randomized controlled trial. Behav Res Ther 2012;50(12):814–21.

33. Argoff C. The coexistence of neuropathic pain, sleep, and psychiatric disorders: a novel treatment approach. Clin J Pain 2007;23:15–22.

34. Roehrs T, Roth T. Sleep and pain: interaction of two vital functions. Semin Neurol 2005;25(1):106–16.

35. Wilson KG, Eriksson MY, D'Eon JL, et al. Major depression and insomnia in chronic pain. Clin J Pain 2002;18:77–83.

36. Rosenthal M, Moore P, Groves E, et al. Sleep improves when patients with chronic OA pain are managed with morning dosing of once a day extended-release morphine sulfate (AVINZA): findings from a pilot study. J Opioid Manag 2007;3(3):145–54.

37. Shaw IR, Lavigne G, Mayer P, et al. Acute intravenous administration of morphine perturbs sleep architecture in healthy pain-free young adults: a preliminary study. Sleep 2005;28(6):677–82.

38. Rosenberg J. Sleep disturbances after non-cardiac surgery. Sleep Med Rev 2001;5(2):129–37.

39. Cheatle MD, Savage SR. Informed consent in opioid therapy: a potential obligation and opportunity. J Pain Symptom Manage 2012;44(1):105–16.

40. Buysse DJ. Insomnia. JAMA 2013;309:706–16.

41. Roehrs T, Roth T. Insomnia pharmacotherapy. Neurotherapeutics 2012;9:728–38.

42. NIH State-of-the-science conference statement on manifestations and management of chronic insomnia in adults. NIH Consens State Sci Statements 2005;22(2):1–30.

43. Bartusch SL, Sanders BJ, D'Alessio JG, et al. Clonazepam for the treatment of lancinating phantom limb pain. Clin J Pain 1996;12:59–62.

44. Menefee LA, Cohen MJ, Anderson WR, et al. Sleep disturbance and nonmalignant chronic pain: a comprehensive review of the literature. Pain Med 2000;1:156–72.

45. King S, Strain J. Benzodiazepine use by chronic pain patients. Clin J Pain 1990;6(2):143–7.

46. Glass J, Lanctôt KL, Herrmann N, et al. Sedative hypnotics in older people with insomnia: meta-analysis of risks and benefits. BMJ 2005;331:1169.

47. Roehrs T, Zorick FJ, Sicklesteel JM, et al. Effects of hypnotics on memory. J Clin Psychopharmacol 1983;3:310–3.

48. Licata SC, Rowlett JK. Abuse and dependence liability of benzodiazepine-type drugs: GABA(A) receptor modulation and beyond. Pharmacol Biochem Behav 2008;90(1):74–89.

49. Pollack M, Kinrys G, Krystal A, et al. Eszopiclone co-administered with escitalopram in patients with insomnia and comorbid generalized anxiety disorder. Arch Gen Psychiatry 2008;65:551–62.

50. Randall S, Roehrs TA, Roth T. Efficacy of eight months of nightly zolpidem: a prospective placebo-controlled study. Sleep 2012;35:1551–7.

51. Roth T, Walsh JK, Krystal A, et al. An evaluation of the efficacy and safety of eszopiclone over 12 months in patients with chronic primary insomnia. Sleep Med 2005;6:487–95.

52. Moldofsky H, Lue FA, Mously C, et al. The effect of zolpidem in patients with fibromyalgia: a dose ranging, double blind, placebo controlled, modified crossover study. J Rheumatol 1996;23:529–33.

53. Roth T, Price JM, Amato DA, et al. The effect of eszopiclone in patients with insomnia and coexisting rheumatoid arthritis: a pilot study. Prim Care Companion J Clin Psychiatry 2009;11:292–301.

54. Mason M, Cates CJ, Smith I. Effects of opioid, hypnotic and sedating medications on sleep-disordered breathing in adults with obstructive sleep apnoea. Cochrane Database Syst Rev 2015;(7):CD011090.

55. Darke S, Deady M, Duflou J. Toxicology and characteristics of deaths involving zolpidem in New South Wales, Australia 2001-2010. J Forensic Sci 2012; 57(5):1259–62.

56. Mayers AG, Baldwin DS. Antidepressants and their effect on sleep. Hum Psychopharmacol 2005;20: 533–59.

57. Moulin DE, Clark AJ, Gilron I, et al. Pharmacological management of chronic neuropathic pain - consensus statement and guidelines from the Canadian Pain Society. Pain Res Manag 2007;12(1):13–21.

58. Shipley JE, Kupfer DJ, Griffin SJ, et al. Comparison of effects of desipramine and amitriptyline on EEG sleep of depressed patients. Psychopharmacology (Berl) 1985;85:14–22.

59. Sonntag A, Rothe B, Guldner J, et al. Trimipramine and imipramine exert different effects on the sleep EEG and on nocturnal hormone secretion during treatment of major depression. Depression 1996;4: 1–13.

60. Gursky JT, Krahn LE. The effects of antidepressants on sleep: a review. Harv Rev Psychiatry 2000;8:298–306.

61. Boyle J, Eriksson ME, Gribble L, et al. Randomized, placebo-controlled comparison of amitriptyline, duloxetine, and pregabalin in patients with chronic diabetic peripheral neuropathic pain: impact on pain, polysomnographic sleep, daytime functioning, and quality of life. Diabetes Care 2012;35:2451–8.

62. Häuser W, Petzke F, Üçeyler N, et al. Comparative efficacy and acceptability of amitriptyline, duloxetine and milnacipran in fibromyalgia syndrome: a systematic review with meta-analysis. Rheumatology (Oxford) 2011;50:532–43.

63. McQuay HJ, Carroll D, Glynn CJ. Dose-response for analgesic effect of amitriptyline in chronic pain. Anaesthesia 1993;48:281–5.

64. McCall C, McCall WV. What is the role of sedating antidepressants, antipsychotics, and anticonvulsants in the management of insomnia? Curr Psychiatry Rep 2012;14(5):494–502.

65. Godfrey RG. A guide to the understanding and use of tricyclic antidepressants in the overall management of fibromyalgia and other chronic pain syndromes. Arch Intern Med 1996;156: 1047–52.

66. Rosenbaum JF. Handbook of psychiatric drug therapy (Google eBook). Philadelphia: Lippincott Williams & Wilkins; 2009. p. 304.

67. Bossini L, Casolaro I, Koukouna D, et al. Off-label uses of trazodone: a review. Expert Opin Pharmacother 2012;13(12):1707–17.

68. Morillas-Arques P, Rodriguez-Lopez CM, Molina-Barea R, et al. Trazodone for the treatment of fibromyalgia: an open-label, 12-week study. BMC Musculoskelet Disord 2010;11:204.

69. Wilson RC. The use of low-dose trazodone in the treatment of painful diabetic neuropathy. J Am Podiatr Med Assoc 1999;89:468–71.

70. Walsh JK, Erman M, Erwin CW, et al. Subjective hypnotic efficacy of trazodone and zolpidem in DSMIII-R primary insomnia. Hum Psychopharmacol 1998; 13:191–8.

71. Kim S-W, Shin I-S, Kim J-M, et al. Effectiveness of mirtazapine for nausea and insomnia in cancer patients with depression. Psychiatry Clin Neurosci 2008;62:75–83.

72. Bendtsen L, Jensen R. Mirtazapine is effective in the prophylactic treatment of chronic tension-type headache. Neurology 2004;62:1706–11.

73. Christodoulou C, Douzenis A, Moussas G, et al. Effectiveness of mirtazapine in the treatment of postherpetic neuralgia. J Pain Symptom Manage 2010; 39:e3–6.

74. Nutt D, Law J. Treatment of cluster headache with mirtazapine. Headache 1999;39:586–7.

75. Calandre EP, Rico-Villademoros F. The role of antipsychotics in the management of fibromyalgia. CNS Drugs 2012;26:135–53.

76. Krymchantowski AV, Jevoux C, Moreira PF. An open pilot study assessing the benefits of quetiapine for the prevention of migraine refractory to the combination of atenolol, nortriptyline, and flunarizine. Pain Med 2010;11:48–52.

77. Backonja M, Beydoun A, Edwards KR, et al. Gabapentin for the symptomatic treatment of painful neuropathy in patients with diabetes mellitus: a randomized controlled trial. JAMA 1998;280: 1831–6.

78. Sabatowski R, Gálvez R, Cherry DA, et al. Pregabalin reduces pain and improves sleep and mood

disturbances in patients with post-herpetic neuralgia: results of a randomised, placebo-controlled clinical trial. Pain 2004;109:26–35.

79. Mula M, Pini S, Cassano GB. The role of anticonvulsant drugs in anxiety disorders: a critical review of the evidence. J Clin Psychopharmacol 2007;27: 263–72.

80. Sateia MJ, Kirby-Long P, Taylor JL. Efficacy and clinical safety of ramelteon: an evidence-based review. Sleep Med Rev 2008;12:319–32.

81. Wilhelmsen M, Amirian I, Reiter RJ, et al. Analgesic effects of melatonin: a review of current evidence from experimental and clinical studies. J Pineal Res 2011;51:270–7.

UNITED STATES POSTAL SERVICE ® Statement of Ownership, Management, and Circulation (All Periodicals Publications Except Requester Publications)

1. Publication Title	2. Publication Number	3. Filing Date
SLEEP MEDICINE CLINICS	025 – 053	9/18/2016

4. Issue Frequency	5. Number of Issues Published Annually	6. Annual Subscription Price
MAR, JUN, SEP, DEC	4	$195.00

7. Complete Mailing Address of Known Office of Publication (Not printer) (Street, city, county, state, and ZIP+4®)

ELSEVIER INC.
360 PARK AVENUE SOUTH
NEW YORK, NY 10010-1710

Contact Person
STEPHEN R. BUSHING

Telephone (Include area code)
215-239-3688

8. Complete Mailing Address of Headquarters or General Business Office of Publisher (Not printer)

ELSEVIER INC.
360 PARK AVENUE SOUTH
NEW YORK, NY 10010-1710

9. Full Names and Complete Mailing Addresses of Publisher, Editor, and Managing Editor (Do not leave blank)

Publisher (Name and complete mailing address)

ADRIANNE BRIGIDO, ELSEVIER INC.
1600 JOHN F KENNEDY BLVD. SUITE 1800
PHILADELPHIA, PA 19103-2899

Editor (Name and complete mailing address)

KATIE PFAFF, ELSEVIER INC.
1600 JOHN F KENNEDY BLVD. SUITE 1800
PHILADELPHIA, PA 19103-2899

Managing Editor (Name and complete mailing address)

PATRICK MANLEY, ELSEVIER INC.
1600 JOHN F KENNEDY BLVD. SUITE 1800
PHILADELPHIA, PA 19103-2899

10. Owner (Do not leave blank. If the publication is owned by a corporation, give the name and address of the corporation immediately followed by the names and addresses of all stockholders owning or holding 1 percent or more of the total amount of stock. If not owned by a corporation, give the names and addresses of the individual owners. If owned by a partnership or other unincorporated firm, give its name and address as well as those of each individual owner. If the publication is published by a nonprofit organization, give its name and address.)

Full Name	Complete Mailing Address
WHOLLY OWNED SUBSIDIARY OF REED/ELSEVIER, US HOLDINGS	1600 JOHN F KENNEDY BLVD. SUITE 1800 PHILADELPHIA, PA 19103-2899

11. Known Bondholders, Mortgagees, and Other Security Holders Owning or Holding 1 Percent or More of Total Amount of Bonds, Mortgages, or Other Securities. If none, check box → ☐ None

Full Name	Complete Mailing Address
N/A	

12. Tax Status (For completion by nonprofit organizations authorized to mail at nonprofit rates) (Check one)
The purpose, function, and nonprofit status of this organization and the exempt status for federal income tax purposes:
☐ Has Not Changed During Preceding 12 Months
☐ Has Changed During Preceding 12 Months (Publisher must submit explanation of change with this statement)

13. Publication Title	14. Issue Date for Circulation Data Below
SLEEP MEDICINE CLINICS	JUNE 2016

PS Form 3526, July 2014 [Page 1 of 4 (see instructions page 4)] PSN: 7530-01-000-9931 PRIVACY NOTICE: See our privacy policy on www.usps.com.

---

13. Publication Title			14. Issue Date for Circulation Data Below
SLEEP MEDICINE CLINICS			JUNE 2016

15. Extent and Nature of Circulation			Average No. Copies Each Issue During Preceding 12 Months	No. Copies of Single Issue Published Nearest to Filing Date
a. Total Number of Copies (Net press run)			351	407
b. Paid Circulation (By Mail and Outside the Mail)	(1)	Mailed Outside-County Paid Subscriptions Stated on PS Form 3541 (Include paid distribution above nominal rate, advertiser's proof copies, and exchange copies)	205	253
	(2)	Mailed In-County Paid Subscriptions Stated on PS Form 3541 (Include paid distribution above nominal rate, advertiser's proof copies, and exchange copies)	0	0
	(3)	Paid Distribution Outside the Mails Including Sales Through Dealers and Carriers, Street Vendors, Counter Sales, and Other Paid Distribution Outside USPS®	32	40
	(4)	Paid Distribution by Other Classes of Mail Through the USPS (e.g., First-Class Mail®)	0	0
c. Total Paid Distribution (Sum of 15b (1), (2), (3), and (4))			237	293
d. Free or Nominal Rate Distribution (By Mail and Outside the Mail)	(1)	Free or Nominal Rate Outside-County Copies included on PS Form 3541	45	54
	(2)	Free or Nominal Rate In-County Copies included on PS Form 3541	0	0
	(3)	Free or Nominal Rate Copies Mailed at Other Classes Through the USPS (e.g., First-Class Mail)	0	0
	(4)	Free or Nominal Rate Distribution Outside the Mail (Carriers or other means)	0	0
e. Total Free or Nominal Rate Distribution (Sum of 15d (1), (2), (3) and (4))			45	54
f. Total Distribution (Sum of 15c and 15e)			282	347
g. Copies not Distributed (See Instructions to Publishers #4 (page #3))			69	60
h. Total (Sum of 15f and g)			351	407
i. Percent Paid (15c divided by 15f times 100)			84%	84%

* If you are claiming electronic copies, go to line 16 on page 3. If you are not claiming electronic copies, skip to line 17 on page 3.

16. Electronic Copy Circulation	Average No. Copies Each Issue During Preceding 12 Months	No. Copies of Single Issue Published Nearest to Filing Date
a. Paid Electronic Copies ▶	0	0
b. Total Paid Print Copies (Line 15c) + Paid Electronic Copies (Line 16a) ▶	237	293
c. Total Print Distribution (Line 15f) + Paid Electronic Copies (Line 16a) ▶	282	347
d. Percent Paid (Both Print & Electronic Copies) (16b divided by 16c × 100) ▶	84%	84%

☒ I certify that 50% of all my distributed copies (electronic and print) are paid above a nominal price.

17. Publication of Statement of Ownership
☒ If the publication is a general publication, publication of this statement is required. Will be printed in the DECEMBER 2016 issue of this publication. ☐ Publication not required.

18. Signature and Title of Editor, Publisher, Business Manager, or Owner

STEPHEN R. BUSHING - INVENTORY DISTRIBUTION CONTROL MANAGER

Date 9/18/2016

I certify that all information furnished on this form is true and complete. I understand that anyone who furnishes false or misleading information on this form or who omits material or information requested on the form may be subject to criminal sanctions (including fines and imprisonment) and/or civil sanctions (including civil penalties).

PS Form 3526, July 2014 (Page 3 of 4) PRIVACY NOTICE: See our privacy policy on www.usps.com

Moving?

Make sure your subscription moves with you!

To notify us of your new address, find your **Clinics Account Number** (located on your mailing label above your name), and contact customer service at:

Email: journalscustomerservice-usa@elsevier.com

800-654-2452 (subscribers in the U.S. & Canada)
314-447-8871 (subscribers outside of the U.S. & Canada)

Fax number: 314-447-8029

Elsevier Health Sciences Division
Subscription Customer Service
3251 Riverport Lane
Maryland Heights, MO 63043

*To ensure uninterrupted delivery of your subscription, please notify us at least 4 weeks in advance of move.

Moving?

Make sure your subscription moves with you!

To notify us of your new address, find your Clinics Account Number (located on your mailing label above your name), and contact customer service at:

Email: journalscustomerservice-usa@elsevier.com

800-654-2452 (subscribers in the U.S. & Canada)
314-447-8871 (subscribers outside of the U.S. & Canada)

Fax number: 314-447-8029

Elsevier Health Sciences Division
Subscription Customer Service
3251 Riverport Lane
Maryland Heights, MO 63043

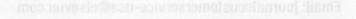

Printed and bound by CPI Group (UK) Ltd, Croydon, CR0 4YY

03/10/2024

01040298-0009